THE URBANA FREE LIBRARY

3 1230 0074 8479

Say Goodbye to Varicose and Spider Veins Now! VERY CLEARLY AND INTELLIGENTLY explains the venous insufficiency disease process, the revolutionary new treatment options available today, and the results patients should and should not expect after treatment. It is an excellent overview of the field of modern venous medicine that will be equally valuable to prospective patients and referring physicians.

Norman Bein, MD, FACS
Board-Certified Surgeon and RVT
Missouri Baptist Medical Center
Vein Specialties, LLC
St. Louis, MO

D1452813

VEIN DISEASE AFFECTS A LARGE P(

the treatments were often wor:

The Urbana Free Library

To renew materials call
217-367-4057

and the medical profession are

exist for treating these common

Dr. Martin does an excellent

patients and physicians. I have treated thousands of patients with vein disease, and I learned new things by reading this book. Written in an easy and clear style, *Say Goodbye to Varicose and Spider Veins Now!* will go a long way toward helping patients understand vein disease and the state-of-the-art treatments available today.

Marcus A. Jimenez, MD, FACS
Indiana Vein and Laser Cente:
Fort Wayne, IN

DR. MARTIN HAS DONE AN (

of venous disease and pu

I am truly impressed at tl

tin's ability to write it wit

this book to anyone wh(

Douglas R. Stafford, MD
Medical Director
Vein Clinics Northwest
Coeur d'Alene, ID

DATE DUE

MAY 24 2011
JUN 27 2011
SEP 06 2011
SEP 29 2011
SEP 23 2011
OCT 01 2011
DEC 06 2012

Rapid advances in the non-invasive treatment of spider and varicose veins have created tremendous benefits to patients, but they also have generated quite a bit of confusion. Overwhelmed with information from the web and other sources, patients often have difficulty sorting fact from "marketing" fiction. Consequently, they are unable to talk intelligently with physicians about treatment options.

I heartily recommend Dr. Martin's outstanding book for anyone who suffers from varicose or spider veins, and for doctors, as well, who want to help educate their patients and themselves about the state-of-the-art treatment options that are available today.

Armen Roupenian, MD, FACS
Medical Director
Vein & Laser Center of New England
Plymouth, MA

Say Goodbye to Varicose and Spider Veins Now! expertly describes the pathophysiology of venous disease and answers common questions that patients have about the disease process and treatment options. It provides specific information about state-of-the-art procedures in understandable language that will help patients choose the treatment options and the medical practitioners that are best for them.

Kara Easton, MS, APN, ANP-C
Northwestern Medical Faculty Foundation
Northwestern Memorial Hospital
Chicago, IL

Venous disease affects more people than heart or peripheral vessel disease, but is under-diagnosed, under-treated, and very misunderstood by medical professionals. This concise and clearly written book gives patients helpful knowledge and guidance to resolve their problems with painful legs. For medical professionals, it provides valuable information and dispels common misperceptions about modern treatment methods. I highly recommend *Say Goodbye to Varicose & Spider Veins Now!*

John Flanagan, MD, FACS
Boarded Vascular Surgery and General Surgery
Founding Physician, Delaware Valley Vein Center
Past President, Delaware Valley Vascular Society of Philadelphia
Philadelphia, PA

IN *SAY GOODBYE TO VARICOSE & SPIDER VEINS NOW!*, GREG MARTIN, MD, DESCRIBES venous diseases and treatments in a straightforward, easy-to-understand manner. This book will be a valuable resource for individuals wishing to make an informed choice about treatment options. It will also serve as an ideal reference for medical professionals who are unfamiliar with the latest techniques in the treatment of venous disease.

I was very impressed with the detailed information contained in every chapter of this excellent book. The personal stories and cartoon depictions add to the enjoyment of the reading experience.

Peggy Bush, APN, CNS, MSN
Midwest Vein & Laser Center
Dayton, OH

ONE OF THE BIGGEST PROBLEMS I FREQUENTLY ENCOUNTER IN MY PRACTICE OF vein medicine is the tremendous amount of misinformation that exists, not only amongst the general public, but also within the medical community. Sadly, many people are completely unaware of the advanced, minimally invasive techniques that are available today for treating venous disease safely, quickly and effectively.

I constantly encounter patients who are being told they will just have to live with their vein problems, or that all they can do is wear compression stockings, or that their only option is to have one of those painful, traumatic vein-stripping procedures that are now considered obsolete. Unfortunately, patients still hear these comments even from their family physicians. None of these things could be further from the truth.

Dr. Greg Martin has done an exceptional job of displacing these false notions with accurate facts about vein disease and today's methods for treating it. *Say Goodbye to Varicose & Spider Veins Now!* is very clear, concise, understandable, and enjoyable to read. It promises to be an outstanding learning tool for the general public and a valuable resource for medical professionals.

Craig I. Schwartz, DO, RVT, RPVI, FACOS, FICS
Medical Director
Vein Centers for Excellence of Kansas City & La Jolie Spa
Kansas City, MO

As a registered nurse, I devote considerable time to educating patients and doctors about the causes and cures of vein disease. I'm always looking for comprehensive, clearly written educational tools, and Dr. Martin's book superbly satisfies that need. *Say Goodbye to Varicose and Spider Veins Now!* gets my highest recommendation!

Maria Bein, RN
Vein Specialties
St. Louis, MO

Say Goodbye to Varicose & Spider Veins Now! will help people who suffer from venous disease make more informed decisions about care. And it will serve as a valuable resource for referring physicians who want to know more about the recent advances in treating vein disease. Packed with useful information and absolutely enjoyable to read, this is a fantastic book!

Kandy Hammond, RN
Varicose Vein Consulting
Dayton, OH

Say Goodbye to Varicose and Spider Veins Now! is a practical, easy-to-read resource about vein disease and the advanced treatment modalities available today. If you suffer from varicose or spider veins, or if you're a physician who refers people who have venous insufficiency problems, you need to read this excellent book!

Tim Ryan, MD, FACS
Medical Director, Lake County Vein Center
Gurnee, IL

GREG MARTIN, MD

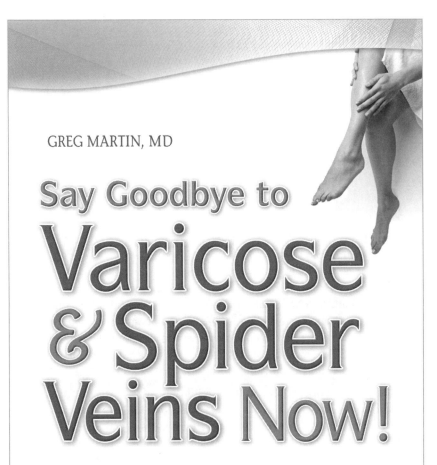

Say Goodbye to
Varicose
& Spider
Veins Now!

How Revolutionary New Medical Techniques
Can Improve Your Health and Quality of Life
by Eliminating Pain, Swelling, Cramps,
Restlessness and Unsightliness in Your Legs

Plentiful Publishing • Brunswick, GA

©2011 Gregory Martin

PLENTIFUL PUBLISHING

650 Scranton Road, Suite C

Brunswick, Georgia 31520

This book is published for general reference. It is not intended to give medical advice, and it should not be relied upon for making medical decisions. Readers should consult their own physician concerning their health needs and questions. The publisher and author disclaim any personal liability, directly or indirectly, for advice or information presented within. Although we have prepared this manuscript with utmost care and diligence and have made every effort to ensure the accuracy and completeness of the information contained within, we assume no responsibility for errors, inaccuracies, omissions, or inconsistencies.

This publication may not be reproduced or transmitted in whole or in part, in any form or by any means, electronic or mechanical, including photocopying, recording, or by an information storage and retrieval system—with the exception of a reviewer who may quote brief passages for a review to be printed in a newspaper, magazine, or e-zine—without the prior written permission of Plentiful Publishing, 650 Scranton Road, Suite C, Brunswick, Georgia 31520.

Martin, Gregory.

Say goodbye to your varicose and spider veins now: how revolutionary new medical techniques can improve your health and quality of life by eliminating pain, swelling, cramps, restlessness, and unsightliness in your legs/Gregory Martin

1st ed. 2011

Library of Congress Control Number: 2010943324

ISBN: 978-0-9831859-0-1

1. Health/fitness 2. Beauty 3. Medical General

All rights reserved

Printed in the United States of America

With great pleasure I dedicate this book to
my gorgeous wife, Terri, who increasingly owns my heart;
my daughter, Felder Anne, who increasingly makes me proud;
and our awesome Creator, whose marvelous
handiwork increasingly fills me with awe.

Contents

I. Varicose and Spider Veins

Chapter One

II. Spider Veins: Diagnoses, Causes, and Treatments

III. Varicose Veins: Diagnoses, Causes, and Treatments

Acknowledgments

Writing a book is truly a collaborative effort, and I want to acknowledge a few of the men and women who made this book possible.

Several noted medical professionals have contributed significantly to my knowledge of vein medicine. Ronald Bush, MD, is one of the world's foremost authorities on the treatment of varicose and spider veins, and a respected pioneer and educator in many of the techniques I describe in this book. For many years I have been fortunate to have him as my close friend and most important mentor.

Kandy Hammond, RN, who practices with Dr. Bush, also has had a strong positive influence on my professional development. I am especially grateful for the support Kandy gave my staff and me as I launched my own vein centers.

John J. Bergen, MD, is truly one of the giants in American vascular surgery and venous medicine, with hundreds of articles, papers, and books to his credit. *The Vein Book,* which he edited, has become one of the most important references for venous practitioners worldwide. I will always value the contributions he made to my career and my life while I was a surgery resident at Northwestern University in Chicago.

I would also like to acknowledge David L. Narhwold, MD, for the confidence and inspiration he imparted to me when I was in surgical training and he was the Chairman of the Department of Surgery at Northwestern University.

Marion Anderson, MD, who was the Chairman of the Department of Surgery when I attended the Medical University of South Carolina in Charleston, was a wonderful teacher, mentor, and friend. A profound influence on me during my medical school years, he was the role model who inspired me to become a surgeon.

I could not have written and published this book without the dedicated efforts of my talented "publishing team." My writer and editor, Michael J. Dowling (*www.MichaelJDowling.com*) made this endeavor not only possible, but enjoyable. In addition to providing professional assistance during the writing process, he expertly shepherded me through the myriad decisions involved with the publication, distribution, and marketing of my book. Mike and his wife, Sarah, also created the book's cartoons.

Tamara and Tom Dever, Monica Thomas, and Erin Stark at TLC Graphics (*www.TLCGraphics.com*) did an outstanding job designing the cover and laying out the interior of the book. On top of producing work of exceptional quality, they are a pleasure to work with.

Carol Capers of Columbus, Georgia, created the excellent medical illustrations. Way to go, Carol!

I've also been blessed with an expert marketing crew:

- Nettie Hartsock of the Hartsock Agency (*www.nettiehartstock.com*) has done a superb job telling the online community about my book.

- Hampton Ryan of Ryan Media Strategies (*www.ryanmediastrategies.com*) proficiently spread the word to traditional media and the book industry.

- Marianne Bohr of Marianne C. Bohr Consulting (*www.mariannecbohr.com*) provided me with valuable publishing and marketing advice and capably handled special sales of my book.

- Michel Linehan of Marketing Alchemy (*www.marketing-alchemy.com*) has worked wonders with my website, *www.GregMartinMD.com*.

My sincere appreciation also goes out to my dedicated staff at the Coastal Georgia Vein Center in Brunswick and the South Georgia Vein Center in Valdosta. Patients continually comment about the warmth and quality of their professional care. Their competent and faithful assistance makes practicing vein medicine a joy.

I also would like to thank my parents, David and Joyce Martin of Easley, SC, for providing such a loving and supportive upbringing, and to extend my appreciation to my in-laws, Dr. Emory and Mikell Linder, for their friendship, love, and support.

Finally, I want to thank my beautiful bride, Terri, and daughter, Felder Anne, for being so supportive and patient with me at all times, but particularly during the past several months as I devoted time to my "Saturday morning book project."

Foreword

by Ronald Bush, MD, FACS

I CONSIDER IT AN HONOR TO BE ASKED TO WRITE THE FOREWORD FOR this excellent book by my friend and colleague, Dr. Greg Martin. I have known Greg for many years. I'm familiar with his work, and I know firsthand that he is an excellent, excellent physician. He is well-versed in the field of endovenous medicine, and he is superbly qualified to write this much-needed publication.

Venous disease affects more than 80 million people in the United States alone. It is a debilitating, painful, and often embarrassing malady that can even be life-threatening.

The good news is that in the past ten years enormous strides have been made in the treatment of chronic venous insufficiency. The bad news is that the vast majority of people who have varicose and spider veins don't know about these new medical advances. Consequently, they needlessly continue to suffer.

To compound the problem, many primary care physicians, dermatologists, and other medical professionals are not fully informed about the new state-of-the-art techniques either. That's not their fault. The new methodologies weren't even in existence when most physicians practicing today were undergoing medical training.

That's why Dr. Martin's book is so important. *Say Goodbye to Varicose & Spider Veins Now!* provides information patients need to make intelligent decisions about their treatment options, and it gives physicians the information they need to make informed referrals.

This useful resource strikes an excellent balance. On one hand, it comprehensively and intelligently presents a wealth of information about the causes of venous disease and the various treatment techniques. At the same time, however, it is written in a style that is easy to understand and enjoyable to read.

Dr. Martin has provided a valuable service by writing this book. I hope and believe it will find a wide audience among patients who suffer from venous disease and medical professionals who refer patients for treatment.

Ronald Bush, MD, FACS
Medical Director, Midwest Vein & Laser Center
Medical Director, Vein Affiliates
Dayton, OH

Foreword

by Jose I. Almeida, MD, FACS

WHAT A PRIVILEGE IT IS TO BE INVITED TO WRITE A FOREWORD FOR DR. Martin's outstanding book! As a fellowship-trained, double-board-certified vascular surgeon, I've been disappointed by the lack of accurate, up-to-date information about treatments for vein disease. *Say Goodbye to Varicose & Spider Veins Now!* superbly fills a vital need.

This book is an excellent primer for lay people and physicians who want to know about the elegant options available today for treating varicose and spider veins. I hope it also will help insurance companies and third-party payers align their policies with the realities of modern venous medicine, so their decisions are more supportive of patients and doctors.

I thoroughly enjoyed reading *Say Goodbye to Varicose & Spider Veins Now!* It's comprehensive, well-documented, well-written, and easy to understand. The clear and attractive illustrations and photographs, real-life patient vignettes, and humorous cartoons add to the reading experience.

Vascular surgery (both arteries and veins) has been my specialty for many years, and since 2002 I've treated venous disease exclusively. I currently chair the International Vein Congress (IVC), which is the largest dedicated annual vein meeting in the world. I've experienced firsthand the paradigm shift that has occurred in the field of venous surgery in the past ten years.

The old vein-stripping operations that were once the standard of care will soon be obsolete. That's a good thing, because they are traumatic, are performed in an operating room under general anesthesia, and require long recovery periods. Furthermore, they weren't all that effective.

But here's the good news: Thanks to the advent of ultrasound, laser, radiofrequency, and other technologies, venous disease can now be treated in the doctor's office under local anesthesia with virtually no pain. The recovery times are short and the results are remarkably better than those achieved by the "big and ugly" procedures of prior years.

Unfortunately, too few people have heard this good news. That's why Dr. Greg Martin's book is so important. I'm proud to be a small part of such a noble endeavor.

Jose I. Almeida, MD, FACS
Medical Director, Miami Vein Center
Founder, International Vein Congress

Introduction

Say Goodbye to Varicose & Spider Veins Now!

IF YOU HAVE VARICOSE VEINS OR SPIDER VEINS, I'VE GOT GOOD NEWS FOR you! No, I'm not glad you have these problems. In fact, I want to help you say goodbye to them. But the good news is that your timing couldn't be better.

In the past ten to fifteen years, medical researchers have achieved extraordinary breakthroughs in the treatment of vein disease. This means that if you're one of the approximately 80 million Americans who suffer from varicose or spider veins, you can now live a happier and healthier life.

Don't be surprised if you haven't heard about these revolutionary medical advances. Most other people, including many members of the medical profession, aren't aware of them either. A huge awareness gap exists, in large part because these major developments have occurred so recently and so suddenly.

Due to this awareness gap, many people with varicose and spider veins needlessly continue to suffer. Perhaps you're one of them. As a physician, I hate to see this. So, I'm writing this book to tell you and others about these dramatic medical breakthroughs.

Even if your vein problems are manageable now, you should find the information contained in this book interesting and valuable. Vein disease is progressive; it gets worse with age. The new state-of-the-art procedures described in these pages make it possible to quickly and economically diagnose and treat vein disease in the early stages. This could help you avoid more serious problems in the future.

Professionals in the dark

Patients are not the only ones who don't know about these revolutionary new treatment methods. Many primary care physicians, physical therapists, nurses, and other health professionals are also impacted by this awareness gap. Consequently, they're not in a position to give the best advice to their patients who have or are at risk of having vein disease.

Over the past twenty-five years, I've performed more than 6,000 varicose vein procedures and tens of thousands of spider vein procedures. I'm aware of the dramatic advances vein medicine has achieved, and I'm tremendously excited about how much better care I can now give my patients. I'm so excited, in fact, that I've undertaken a mission.

A physician on a mission

My mission—indeed, my passion—is to inform the general public, members of the medical profession, and representatives of the media about these revolutionary new treatment techniques. I want the world to know that the majority of new vein problems can now be prevented, and that most existing vein problems can be successfully treated in office settings with much less discomfort, inconvenience, and expense than ever before.

A second aspect of my mission is to clarify some prevailing misconceptions, including the one that vein treatments are invasive, short-lived, debilitating, and expensive. That once was true in many cases. But the medical realities have changed, and I'm on a mission to help spread the word.

Another misperception I want to help dispel is that vein treatments are only for vain people. Many, if not most, vein procedures are medically necessary. Left unattended for a number of years, both spider veins and varicose veins can lead to more serious health problems.

Furthermore, quality-of-life and self-esteem are legitimate health issues. I once erroneously considered vein procedures performed primarily for cosmetic purposes to be a luxury, but no longer. After treating many thousands of patients with all types of vein diseases, I'm keenly aware of the importance of emotional as well as physical health.

The third aspect of my mission is to offer encouragement to you and others who might suffer from vein diseases. You have not been forgotten. Medical researchers have been working diligently to address your concerns, and they've achieved remarkable success.

To overcome the debilitating effects of vein diseases, you no longer need to undergo invasive, expensive treatments of questionable veracity. If you suffer from spider veins or varicose veins, remedies are available that can effectively, efficiently, affordably, and dramatically improve your physical and emotional health.

So that's my mission, and this book is an important part of it. It contains information you can use to help you make better decisions, in conjunction with your physician, about how to prevent, diagnose, and treat vein disease. But before I can expect you to read further, I owe you a brief description of my background.

My credentials

I am a general surgeon certified by the American Board of Surgery and the American Board of Phlebology. The latter board, which was established in 2008, recognizes modern vein medicine and surgery as an important new specialty. I am also a fellow with the American College of Surgeons and a member of the American College of Phlebology.

After earning my Doctor of Medicine degree at the Medical University of South Carolina in Charleston in 1986, I fulfilled my surgery internship and residency requirements from 1986 to 1991 at Northwestern University in Chicago, where I served as chief surgery resident during my final year.

I've been performing vein operations since 1986, initially as one aspect of my training and later in private practice. In the early years, I performed dozens of the old vein-stripping operations.

In 2003, I began studying the new vein medical procedures under Dr. Ron Bush of the Midwest Vein & Laser Center in Dayton, Ohio. Dr. Bush, a pioneer and leading educator in the treatment of vein diseases, is one of the foremost authorities in the field.

In early 2004, I opened a state-of-the-art vein treatment center in South Georgia, and in 2005 I began devoting my full-time energies to treating vein patients. In 2006, I opened a second vein treatment center in Southeast Georgia.

Because I've been among the first wave of physicians utilizing the advanced vein treatment techniques, to the best of my knowledge I'm one of the more experienced physicians in the world in this exciting new specialty. I know firsthand how much better care we can give vein patients today. That's why I see the need for this book and am motivated to write it.

What this book is and isn't

This is not a medical reference book or a scholarly treatise; neither is it intended to offer medical advice or to supplant the role of your physician. My purpose is simply to help close the awareness gap by offering education, clarification, and encouragement.

If you're a patient or prospective patient concerned about vein disease, I hope this book will help you better safeguard and manage your personal health. Should you need to consult a doctor about a vein problem, this book may help you decide how and when.

If you're a healthcare professional, this book can serve as a primer to introduce you to some of the state-of-the-art vein treatments that are now available. This knowledge may enable you to offer better advice and care to your patients who suffer from vein problems.

In the past few years, modern medicine has taken some amazing strides in the treatment of vein disease. What a privilege and pleasure it is to tell you about them.

I like this mission!

Section One

Varicose and Spider Veins

Fact and Fiction

BECAUSE OF THE AWARENESS GAP I REFERRED TO IN THE INTRODUCTION, many people have misperceptions about vein disease. You may be one of them. In this chapter I'll attempt to dispel some of the most common erroneous notions.

Misperception: Leg discomfort is a normal part of aging.

FACT: Pain, heaviness, swelling, or fatigue in the legs is abnormal at any age. However, untreated vein problems do worsen with age because your veins are in a constant battle against two powerful enemies: time and gravity. If you suffer from any of the above symptoms, I encourage you to consult a vein specialist.

Misperception: Vein diseases aren't particularly important or serious.

FACT: Vein diseases are a tremendous health problem. According to the American College of Phlebology, varicose and spider veins affect more than 80 million adult Americans.[1] The burden of venous diseases on society from disability and other effects is almost incalculable.[2] Because of vein disease, it's estimated that in the United States alone more than 4.6 million work days are lost each year.[3]

But that's just the beginning. The most significant burden is borne by the affected individuals and their families.

> Time and gravity are the enemies. That's true of many things in life, but it's especially true of leg veins.

- Patients with varicose veins and venous insufficiency problems run serious long-term risks of blood clot, phlebitis, and pulmonary embolism. These can be life-threatening concerns.

- Leg pain and swelling can cause significant discomfort. In advanced cases, these disabilities can interfere with work and other important aspects of life.

- Venous insufficiency problems seem to be worsening in recent years, especially among women, perhaps because Americans today typically spend less time walking and exercising, and more time sitting at desks, in cars, and in front of televisions. Some medical authorities have labeled the increase in vein disease an epidemic.

- Vein disease can develop into wounds, especially in the lower legs, that can be extremely debilitating and stubborn to treat.

- Vein disease can cause rashes, discoloring of skin, and severe scarring of skin and soft tissue.

- Unsightly vein disease can seriously damage self-esteem and impair quality of life.

Vein disease is vastly under-diagnosed and under-treated. Phlebology—the practice of vein medicine—has traditionally been the overlooked stepchild of medical specialties; it's been called the "Cinderella" of clinical medicine. Even many physicians are unaware of the significance of these health problems.

That's why I'm writing this book. I want to help patients know how to prevent and treat leg-vein problems, and I want to help medical practitioners know when and how to refer patients to specialists.

Misperception: Vein disease treatments are painful and scarring.

FACT: Many of the old methods for treating vein problems were painful, and some left unsightly scars. The vein-stripping procedures previously used to treat varicose veins are one example. The hypertonic-saline injections once used to treat spider veins are another.

But times have changed! The open, invasive vein operations of past years have been superseded by minimally invasive techniques that leave virtually no scars, even in the most advanced cases of varicose veins. And today's procedures—which utilize laser surgery, ultrasound guidance, and other technological advances—entail little discomfort.

Misperception: Vein treatments are often ineffective and short-lived.

FACT: A decade ago vein surgery was indeed far less effective. After treatment for varicose veins, upwards of 85-90 percent of patients experienced a recurrence of the disease sometime during their lifetimes.

Although it's still somewhat true that venous insufficiency can never be completely cured, when procedures are performed by experienced and capable physicians using modern techniques, the statistics are reversed. Instead of a recurrence rate of 90 percent, 90 percent or better of varicose vein patients may never need further treatment.

Similar good news applies to spider veins. Today, a good series of spider vein treatments by an experienced medical practitioner utilizing state-of-the-art techniques can clear 98 percent or more of the disease. And in my experience, such treatments may prevent 85 percent or more of abnormal veins from recurring. The great majority of vein patients have good lifetime benefits, though occasional follow-up treatments should be considered.

Misperception: Vein treatments can actually cause future vein problems.

FACT: Unfortunately, this used to be true. The older treatment methods, which involved the cutting and dividing of veins, could increase the probability of future vein problems. Consequently, it was not unusual to hear patients say, "I had vein treatments, but my veins came back!"

Modern vein procedures attack the root of the problem. They seal off the abnormal veins so they cease to function. To use a gardening analogy, the old methods were like cutting weeds off above ground, and the new methods destroy them at the roots.

Misperception: Vein operations are severely debilitating and require extended recovery periods.

FACT: That was true a few years ago, when most vein operations took place in hospitals under general anesthesia. Typically, patients could not resume their normal activities for four to six weeks. But treatments with today's advanced techniques are almost always performed in the doctor's office using local anesthesia, so most patients can return to work in one to three days. In two to five days, they're able to walk a few miles.

Misperception: Vein surgery is expensive.

FACT: Today's advanced medical procedures are performed in a doctor's office, which means that fees for hospital services, ambulatory surgery-center services, and general anesthesia are eliminated. Costs to insurance companies and patients are decreased by 80 percent or more.

The fee for state-of-the-art spider vein procedures ranges from $200 to $350 for a 30-minute session. Most patients need three to six treatments. Using this range as a guide, the total cost for a complete regimen might run between $600 and $2,100.

Treatments for varicose veins are more expensive than treatments for spider veins. But because they're performed in an office setting, they're considerably less expensive today than they were ten years ago. Furthermore, these costs are usually covered by insurance.

Misperception: Vein treatments are only for vain people.

FACT: When I was a general surgeon and vein surgery was only one aspect of my practice, I used to be somewhat hesitant to treat patients primarily for cosmetic reasons. But over time, as vein surgery became my focus and I saw the debilitating effects vein problems had on self-esteem and quality of life, my opinion changed.

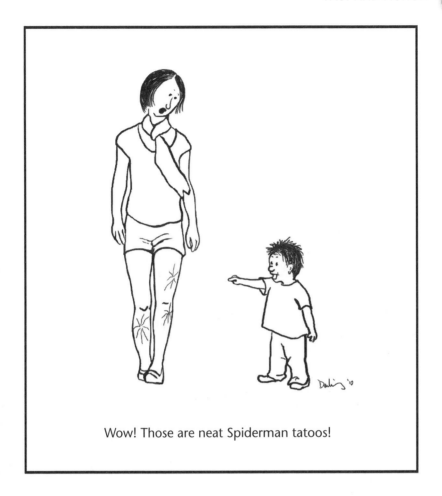

Wow! Those are neat Spiderman tatoos!

I no longer feel the least bit apologetic about performing cosmetic vein treatments. I've seen firsthand how spider veins can curtail lifestyles. I've treated many patients who were too embarrassed to wear shorts, skirts, or sandals, even in the heat of summer.

To illustrate this point, I'll tell you a story about an attractive, 28-year-old teacher we'll call Kathy Smith. One day at recess, a student in her first-grade class said, "Mrs. Smith, your legs look just like my grandma's." Kathy called my office that afternoon to make an appointment.

It turns out that she had rather severe spider veins, especially for such a young person. Her condition probably would have been even more severe if she had given birth to children. The treatment was successful, and I don't think she'll ever hear comments like that again.

Over time, I have grown to appreciate the importance of emotional as well as physical health. My commitment to holistic healing is reaffirmed every time I see how cosmetic procedures can create great value for patients with vein diseases.

Not infrequently, treatments that appear to be cosmetic niceties turn out to be medical necessities. Vein problems are often accompanied by leg pain and swelling, and they can lead to more serious complications, such as blood clots, rashes, and leg wounds.

**Perhaps you now can understand why
I'm so excited about these revolutionary
new medical treatments.**

They've already brought hope and relief to thousands, and millions more stand to benefit from them. In succeeding chapters, I'll give you the information you need to reap these benefits.

---

1. "ACP Patient Information for Vein Treatment." American College of Phlebology, accessed January 12, 2011. http://phlebology.org/patientinfo/index.html.

2. J. Bergan, *The Vein Book* (Oxford, U.K.: Elsevier, 2007), xvii.

3. P.F. Lawrence and C.E. Gazak, "Epidemiology of Chronic Venous Insufficiency" in *Atlas of Endoscopic Perforator Vein Surgery,* eds, P. Gloviczki and J. Bergan (London: Springer-Verlag, 1998), 31-44.

Keeping Your Guard Up

Symptoms and Risk Factors
for Varicose and Spider Veins

SPIDER VEINS ARE VERY SMALL VEINS—ABOUT ONE TO THREE MILLIMETERS in width—that are visible in the top layer (epidermis) of the skin. If your skin is fair, they will tend to be reddish or purplish in color. If your skin is darker, the colors will be less pronounced.

The formal medical term for a spider vein is *telangiectasia*. No wonder most people simply call them spider veins! They probably got that lively moniker because they tend to emanate out from a central cluster, like the legs of a spider.

Over the years, spider veins tend to enlarge (i.e., dilate), take on a beaded appearance, and turn more bluish. The medical term for this advanced condition is *venulectasia*.

Varicose veins are larger veins located just under the surface of the skin. Normally you can't see them, but when they dilate and bulge outward, they're more visible than desired.

Varicose veins are generally a more serious condition than spider veins, but there are plenty of exceptions. I've seen patients with visually severe varicose veins who have few, if any, symptoms. And I've treated patients who have such severe cases of spider veins that they've been classified by physicians or governmental authorities as medically disabled.

Both varicose veins and spider veins result from chronic venous insufficiency, which is the abnormal flow of blood through the veins. Because there is so much overlap between the two—in fact, it's not unusual to have both—we'll discuss their symptoms and warning signs together.

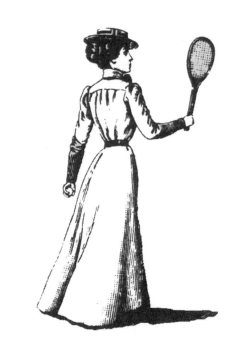

In the good old days,
leg vein problems weren't so noticeable.

Seven symptoms, or warning signs, of chronic venous insufficiency (CVI):

1. The visible presence of varicose veins or spider veins

Both spider veins and varicose veins are frequently visible to the naked eye. That makes this warning sign very straightforward: If you see them, you have them!

2. Leg pain or discomfort

Do you regularly experience aching, heaviness, throbbing, burning, itching, cramping, tingling, stinging, or numbness in your legs, especially after prolonged standing or sitting? There's a good chance this pain or discomfort is caused by CVI.

3. Swollen legs or ankles

Swelling in your legs, especially when it occurs late in the day and is aggravated by prolonged sitting or standing, might indicate CVI. But this warning sign is a bit less reliable. Swelling can also be caused by hormone conditions; various diseases of the heart, liver, or kidneys; and lymphedema, a condition that occurs especially in overweight people when the lymph vessels inadequately drain tissue fluid up the legs.

4. Tired or heavy legs

If your legs suddenly get fatigued after a modest amount of activity or after standing for just a few minutes, you could have CVI. Not infrequently, this fatigue is accompanied by an overall lack of energy.

5. Discoloration and scarring of skin on legs

Rashes, redness, or inflammation of the skin, especially around the lower legs and ankles, can be an indication of vein disease (*venous stasis dermatitis*). Long-standing vein disease may cause brown or dark stains on the skin (*hyperpigmentation*). In advanced cases, the skin and soft tissue around the lower legs and ankles scars so severely that it looks and feels like leather (a condition known as *lipodermatosclerosis*).

6. Open sores or ulcers on the lower legs or ankles

When severe venous insufficiency is allowed to persist for a long period of time, open wounds (*venous stasis ulcers*) can develop. More medical research is needed to pinpoint the cause of this condition, but poor circulation of blood from the veins back to the heart is undoubtedly a contributing factor.

Venous stasis ulcers can be slow to heal. Some of my patients have struggled with this condition for months, even years. The vein ablation treatments that we'll be discussing can accelerate the healing process. More importantly, these treatments substantially lower the risk of ulcer recurrence.

7. Restless legs or cramps in the legs, especially at night

Chronic venous insufficiency can cause an uncomfortable tingling sensation in the legs, especially in the evenings and when retiring at night. Patients with this condition feel compelled to move their legs and are often uncomfortable at rest.

Some recent research seems to link CVI with restless legs syndrome (RLS).[4] Although this correlation is not yet firmly established or broadly accepted in medical circles, my conversations with several researchers cause me to believe that over the next few years we will witness some important advances in the treatment of these two serious quality-of-life issues.

If you suffer from both leg-vein disease and RLS, you might consider having your varicose or spider veins treated before you begin taking medications, such as Requip. I have treated several hundred patients who have had RLS and CVI, and most have achieved substantial relief from both.

Nine factors that increase your risk of contracting leg-vein disease:

Now that you're aware of the symptoms of leg-vein disease, let's talk about a few of the factors that increase your risk of contracting it. In some cases, this information will allow you to modify your behaviors to reduce your risks. In other cases, you may not be able to reduce your risks, but you can at least be more alert.

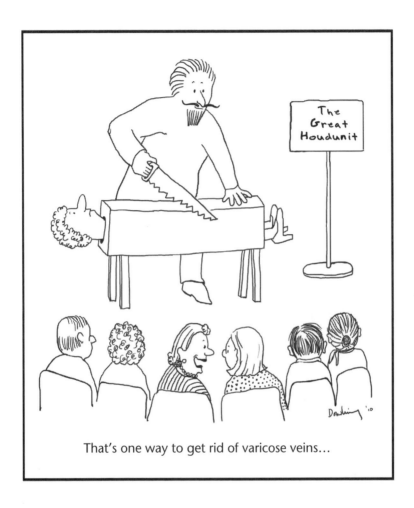

That's one way to get rid of varicose veins...

1. Age

The older you get, the more likely you are to get varicose and spider veins. Not much you can do about that, unfortunately.

2. Family history

It's not quite accurate to say that varicose and spider veins are "all in the family," but genetics certainly does play a contributing role. Of course, it's too late to change your family history, but you can and should be more watchful if vein disease runs in your family.

If either of your parents had varicose or spider veins, you run a greater-than-average risk of having vein problems. If both of your parents had vein disease, your risk is compounded. Sometimes this genetic tendency will skip a generation. Your risk is elevated even if your parents did not suffer from leg-vein disease, but one or more of your four grandparents did.

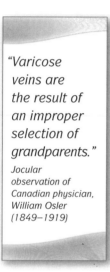

"Varicose veins are the result of an improper selection of grandparents."

Jocular observation of Canadian physician, William Osler (1849–1919)

3. Race

Although people of all races can contract vein disease, it is more commonly found in Caucasians.

4. Gender

Women are almost 2½ times more likely to have vein disease than men. Said another way, approximately 70 percent of people who have varicose or spider vein problems are female, while only 30 percent are male.

5. Multiple pregnancies

Every pregnancy increases the risk and the probable severity of vein disease. I'll discuss this further in chapter 5.

6. A sedentary lifestyle and lack of exercise

Many people who spend a great deal of time sitting or standing throughout their lives never develop vein disease, so this appears to be a less significant risk factor than some others. But if you are genetically prone to venous insufficiency, a sedentary lifestyle may accelerate or aggravate the condition.

As we will discuss in the next chapter, the calf muscles play an important role in pumping the blood through the leg veins back to the heart. People who have active lifestyles that include walking and other forms of exercise tend to have better muscle tone and reduced risk of vein disease. So get off the couch!

7. An occupation or lifestyle that entails prolonged standing, walking, or sitting

Vein problems are more common today than they were one hundred years ago, perhaps in part because people spend so much time standing, working at computers, and riding in cars.

8. An overweight or obese condition

Being overweight or obese is at least a mild risk factor for varicose and spider veins. Obese patients are often more difficult to treat and may have a higher risk of disease recurrence. One reason, some theorize, is that higher abdominal pressure from obesity can interfere with the rising flow of blood through the veins of the legs.

Obese patients also tend to have a higher incidence of swollen legs. However, this is not necessarily due to leg-vein disease. Overweight people frequently have what can be considered lymphedema, which occurs when the lymph vessels fail to adequately drain tissue fluid up the legs. This may be due, at least in part, to the additional bulk in the groin and upper thighs, which can put pressure on the lymph vessels and create a partial blockage.

9. History of leg injury

Patients who have experienced some types of trauma in their legs or ankles can have a higher risk of vein disease. For example, a surgical incision, the impact of a baseball, or the kick of a horse can cause damage that will eventually result in varicose or spider veins.

Minimizing the risk of blood clots

Many physicians who treat vein disease—I among them—think that people with varicose veins have a higher risk of blood-clot problems and phlebitis than people with normal leg veins. Varicose veins create increased pressure in the vein system (*venous hypertension*) and cause the blood flow to be more sluggish. Both of these conditions are known to be risk factors for blood clots, particularly in the legs.

A few blood-clot conditions are rather superficial and benign. For example, superficial thrombophlebitis, a condition involving smaller amounts of blood clots and inflammation in veins just under the skin, tends to be self-limited and will usually resolve with time. Local heat, anti-inflammatory medication, and compression hose (or socks) can also be useful in treatment.

However, in a fraction of patients, blood clots may propagate from the superficial vein system to the deep vein system, which is composed of the larger vessels deep within the muscles of the legs and pelvis. When the body develops this condition, known as deep vein thrombosis (DVT), clots can break off and migrate to and through the right side of the heart, where they can block arteries to the lungs and cause a pulmonary embolism.

The symptoms of DVT are a sudden pain, swelling, or discoloration in one leg. The symptoms of pulmonary embolism may include chest pains, shortness of breath, and unexplained loss of consciousness. DVT and pulmonary embolism are considered medical emergencies that can be health- and life-threatening.

If you have the above conditions, see a physician immediately. And if you have varicose veins, it's advisable to have them treated so as to avoid unnecessary risks.

Now that you know some of the symptoms and risk factors associated with vein disease, it's time to learn what causes it.

---

4. B. McDonagh, T. King, and R.C. Guptan, "Restless Legs Syndrome in Patients with Chronic Venous Disorders: An Untold Story," *Phlebology* 22, no. 4 2007: 156-63.

CHAPTER THREE

Yikes! Where Did These Things Come From?

The Causes of Varicose and Spider Veins

YOU'LL BE BETTER ABLE TO PREVENT AND TREAT SPIDER VEINS AND VARI-cose veins if you understand what causes them. So, let's start with a brief anatomy lesson.

All around your circulatory system

Your circulatory system has two components: your artery system and your vein system. They're completely opposite, yet amazingly complementary (like men and women!).

Your **artery system,** powered by the pumping action of your heart, transports blood at a brisk rate under considerable pressure to the extremities of your body. There, microscopic vessels called capillaries distribute the oxygen and nutrients in your blood to the neighboring tissues through a process called microcirculation. Although arteries are rather small in diameter, their thick, muscular walls equip them to handle the high pressure.

Your **vein system** has an opposite assignment. Its job is to acquire blood containing carbon dioxide and waste products from your capillaries and return it to your heart. From there it goes to your lungs, where it is replenished with oxygen.

> *I praise you because I am fearfully and wonderfully made; your works are wonderful, I know that full well.*
>
> Psalm 139:14

Your vein system is considerably more complex than your artery system. The pressure within your veins is lower than in your arteries—at times it's even negative—and the flow of blood is slower and more passive. It's so passive, in fact, that it can be easily influenced by external factors. For example, when you inhale deeply, your body creates a sort of vacuum that pulls the blood in your veins toward your chest and heart.

Veins have thinner walls than arteries, and they generally have larger diameters and greater storage capacities. There are also many more of them. Your vein system is so large, in fact, that at this very moment it's holding approximately 75 to 80 percent of your body's blood.

Although your vein system operates under low pressure, it has a high-pressure job. It must carry blood up your legs and back to your heart against the force of gravity, and it must accomplish this feat without the help of the heart pump. Talk about a seemingly insurmountable challenge!

Two ingenious features

Our Creator has overcome this challenge by designing into our bodies two ingenious features. The first is called the calf muscle pump (*musculovenous pump*). It utilizes the tone and contraction in your leg muscles to squeeze the blood up through the veins in your legs. Although the muscles in the feet and thighs are important, studies have shown that the calf muscles generate at least 85 percent of the pumping action.

I grew up on a small farm in South Carolina, and I've had a few experiences milking cows. So I sometimes tell my patients that this is the body's way of "milking" the blood back to the heart.

Tone refers to the resting, or baseline, tension of a muscle. It's the amount of pressure a muscle generates in a state of rest. Muscles with good tone produce strong pressures. That's why you should regularly take walks and engage in other types of physical exercise. Strong calf muscles can help prevent vein disease, or at least lessen its severity.

The calf muscle pump by itself is not sufficient to "milk" blood upward through your veins against the force of gravity. So it's a good thing that each of the larger veins in your legs has another ingenious feature that is not present in your arteries.

We call this feature a valve. Valves are very thin, two-leaflet structures that allow blood to flow in only one direction. A healthy valve, as shown in figure 3.1, permits blood to flow up your legs, but not down. When everything is working properly, the pumping action of your muscles will efficiently push blood upward through your veins and back to your heart.

So that's what causes varicose and spider veins!

However, if the valves in your veins become defective as depicted in figure 3.2, blood will begin to flow in the wrong direction (downward). Due to the force of gravity, it will tend to accumulate, or pool, in your lower legs and feet under ever-increasing pressure.

Over time, this pressurized pooling will cause the walls of your veins to become weaker and thinner. It's not uncommon for them to become in-flamed or enlarged (dilated), to bulge out (a symptom of varicose veins, in particular), and to develop scar tissue. Since veins have sensory nerve fibers, this can result in considerable discomfort, especially after prolonged periods of sitting or standing.

All spider and varicose vein problems arise because of leaky valves or other deficiencies within the veins. We call this condition chronic venous insufficiency (CVI).

In a healthy vein system, blood flows steadily and efficiently back to your heart. But if you have chronic venous insufficiency due to leaky vein valves, your blood flow will be abnormally sluggish (a condition called *stasis*). This dramatically increases the risk of blood clots, which are a major hazard to health and life.

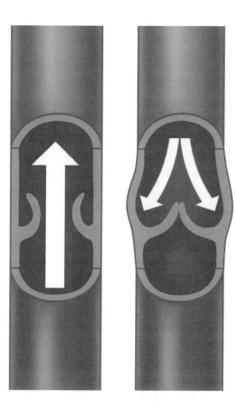

Fig. 3.1 A normally functioning vein valve.

Fig. 3.2 An incompetent vein valve.

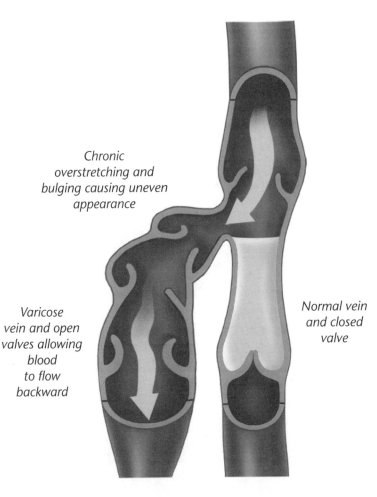

Chronic
overstretching and
bulging causing uneven
appearance

Varicose
vein and open
valves allowing
blood
to flow
backward

Normal vein
and closed
valve

Fig. 3.3 An insufficent,
or incompetent, vein valve
(on the left) and a healthy valve

Three simple steps to relieve leg discomfort

If you have leg-vein problems, here are three quick and easy steps you can take immediately to relieve discomfort in your legs and promote healthier blood flow:

1. Elevate your legs, or simply lie down. This allows gravity to be your friend instead of your enemy.

2. Strengthen your leg muscles through exercise. Your regimen doesn't need to be strenuous; even simple walking is great. Exercise helps relieve symptoms of leg-vein disease and reduces future severity.

3. Use external compression devices to facilitate the flow of blood through your leg veins and help prevent the accumulation of blood in your lower extremities. Some popular devices are compression hose, socks, and wraps.

In the next chapter we'll discuss in more detail some noninvasive techniques for slowing the onset and lessening the severity of spider veins and varicose veins.

Jeannette Gilreath's Story

Jeannette Gilreath, age 70, is a retired kindergarten teacher and an avid clogger.

I've been clogging for twenty-five years. I'm part of a dance group that performs all over the state and even the region. We have to wear short skirts, but I used to be so self-conscious about my spider veins that I would wear darker hose than the other girls. I wouldn't wear shorts or a swimsuit, even around my own swimming pool. I didn't want my own husband to see my legs.

I saw a magazine article that Dr. Martin had written about the new vein treatment methods that have been developed in the last ten years, so I went to see him. The procedures were simple, and Dr. Martin and his staff were great. They made me feel like a real person. We just chatted away while he was treating me.

I've had four or five treatments now, and my legs look so much better! Before, they would itch, and I would get swelling around my left knee, but all that is gone. My legs feel good, and I'm no longer embarrassed to wear shorts.

I tell everybody I know about Dr. Martin. I'm just sorry I didn't have these treatments a long time ago.

Home Improvement

*Conservative Measures for
Preventing and Treating Vein Disease*

WHEN PATIENTS ASK ME WHAT THEY COULD HAVE DONE TO PREVENT vein disease, I say with a grin, "You should have chosen different parents!"

This answer, although partially accurate, isn't much help. It's obviously too late to alter your family history. However, you can indeed take a few steps at home to slow the onset and lessen the severity of spider and varicose veins. In this chapter, we'll discuss three of the most important measures: *elevation, exercise,* and *elastic compression therapy*.

Elevate those legs!

Elevating your legs is one of the best things you can do to promote the healthy flow of blood through your leg veins and to relieve some of the discomfort, swelling, and other symptoms associated with chronic venous insufficiency. But this is easier said than done.

Most footstools, ottomans, and reclining chairs don't elevate your legs and feet high enough to be beneficial. And even though putting your feet up on your desk at work might be good for your vein health, it may not be so good for your career.

Lying down is ideal because it positions your feet close to heart level, but it isn't always practical. A good compromise is to look for opportunities to at least elevate your feet above the level of your hip joints. Even if you have an active lifestyle, you should be able to take intermittent breaks to elevate your legs several times a day.

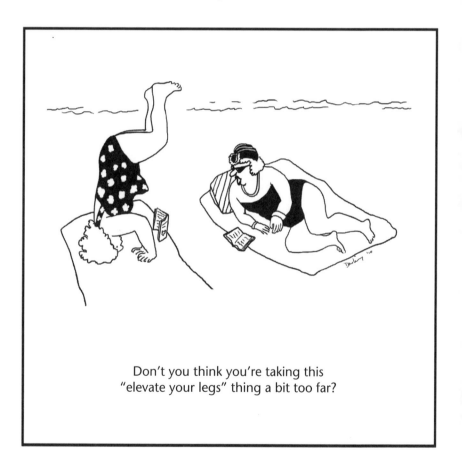

Don't you think you're taking this
"elevate your legs" thing a bit too far?

Get off the couch!

Leg-vein problems seem to have reached epidemic proportions in recent years. I suspect that's partly due to our sedentary modern lifestyles, which make it more difficult to maintain good muscle tone. As I've pointed out, you need regular exercise for well-toned muscles, and you need well-toned muscles in your legs—especially in your calves—for the proper flow of blood through your veins.

When your calf muscles don't pump properly, blood tends to accumulate in your leg veins under increasing pressure. This dramatically increases your chances of getting varicose and spider veins. Exercise reduces these risks by increasing the efficiency of the blood flow in your deep vein system, which in turn decreases the pressure in your superficial vein system.

All types of exercises are good for vein health, especially those that strengthen your calf muscles. Walking is one of the best things you can do. Running, biking, swimming, tennis, golf, weightlifting, and lots of other sports also are excellent.

Don't have time to exercise? My recommendation is to "make" the time. Build exercise into your schedule. Find an accountability partner to exercise with you.

No matter how busy you are, I know you can make time for "toe raises." Throughout the day, strengthen and exercise your calf muscles by simply raising yourself up on the balls of your feet and then lowering yourself back down. Do several of these toe raises whenever you have a few moments. Your leg veins will appreciate it!

Keep the pressure on!

Medical studies have shown that applying compression to the legs can lessen the severity and slow the progression of leg-vein disease. It also promotes healing of leg veins after treatment and provides considerable relief from swelling and other symptoms.

Graduated, elastic compression hose (or socks, as they are often called in the case of men) are the most common method for applying compression. The term "graduated" means that the hose fit more tightly around the feet and ankles, and less tightly higher up the legs, so they push—or "milk"—the venous blood and tissue fluid up the legs.

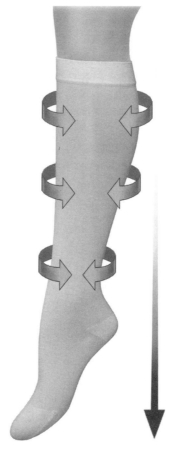

Compression
increases

Get fit!

Compression hose come in three different versions (levels):

- Knee-high hose (or socks) cover to just below the knee.
- Thigh-high hose (or socks) cover to the upper thigh. In my practice, this is the version I prefer to use with patients after treatment.
- Waist-high hose fit essentially like pantyhose.

Some of my patients prefer the waist-high version because they're less likely to slide or roll down the legs. Since they completely cover both legs, however, many people prefer knee-high or thigh-high hose, especially in warmer weather.

To prevent knee-high and thigh-high hose from sliding down your legs, I recommend applying water-soluble skin glue. It's effective, it washes off very easily, it doesn't stain, and it's readily available from most of the companies that market compression hose.

Take your choice!

Compression hose are also available in a variety of grades, colors, and styles. We'll discuss each in turn.

Grade

The grade specifies how much pressure the hose applies. On the product package, pressure is expressed in millimeters of mercury (mm of Hg). The higher the grade, the greater the pressure. Grade-4 hose, for example, have a pressure rating of 40 to 50 mm of Hg, while grade-1 hose have a pressure rating of 20 to 30 mm of Hg.

In the past, many physicians prescribed higher grades of compression hose (grades 2, 3 & 4) because they believed they were more effective. However, higher-grade hose are thicker, less comfortable, less stylish, and more difficult to manipulate. Some people, especially elderly patients with arthritis, liken putting on high-grade hose to a wrestling match.

Fortunately, more recent medical studies and my own clinical experience have shown that grade-1 hose are often sufficient. I prefer them because they're more comfortable and patients are more likely to wear them. Unworn compression hose are worthless.

Color

Color is a matter of preference. From a medical standpoint, no one color is better than another. The most popular colors for compression hose are black, suntan, and natural.

Style

Chose a style of compression hose that gives you the appearance you prefer and the medical support you require. Some hose for women resemble fashion hose, and some of the knee-high and thigh-high socks for men look just like dress socks when worn under slacks or jeans.

Get a prescription, or not!

You can purchase nonprescription compression hose off the shelf at retail stores. If you have only mild symptoms of vein disease, or if you simply want to relieve the pressure on your legs late in the day, these may be adequate.

However, if you have a more severe case of leg-vein disease, I recommend purchasing compression hose by prescription at pharmacies, medical supply stores, online, or from your doctor. High-quality, prescription compression hose are manufactured by a number of different companies (a partial list can be found in appendix C).

Getting a good fit is sometimes a challenge, so I advise buying your hose from your physician, if possible. Most doctors who specialize in the treatment of leg-vein disease offer them for sale in their offices as a service to their patients.

Compress the healing process!

Wearing compression hose for one to two weeks after treatment for varicose or spider veins will accelerate the healing process, sooth the mild tenderness, and limit bruising and inflammation. Following spider vein treatments, they give you more "bang for your buck" by facilitating the clearing of veins.

For maximum effectiveness, compression hose should be worn all day, every day. Apply them as soon as possible after arising in the morning, and leave them on until you retire at night. It's fine to take a break from the hose while sleeping.

If for some reason you decide to defer treatment of leg-vein disease, compression hose can be a helpful bridge remedy to slow disease progression and relieve swelling and other symptoms. However, you will probably find it difficult to wear hose on a daily, indefinite basis because of comfort and style issues. That's why I recommend vein treatment as the preferable long-term option.

Don't get traveler's thrombosis!

Traveler's thrombosis is the colloquial term for acute deep vein thrombosis (DVT) that can develop during long periods of sitting, such as when traveling on a plane or in a car. DVT is a common medical condition in our modern society, and it can be life-threatening (see appendix A).

Patients with chronic venous insufficiency, especially those with varicose veins, have an elevated risk for traveler's thrombosis. Prolonged sitting tends to cause the flow of blood in the legs to become sluggish, which can lead to the development of blood clots in the large deep veins of the legs.

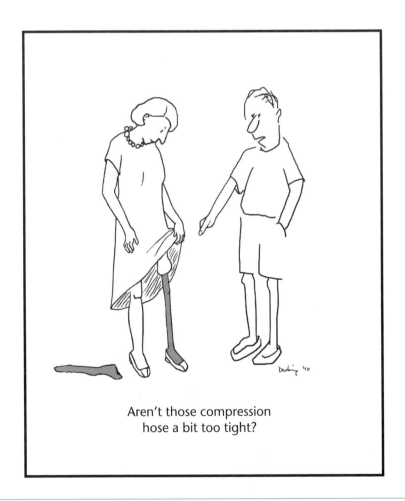

Aren't those compression
hose a bit too tight?

The good news is that traveler's thrombosis is preventable. I advise patients, especially those with varicose veins or leg-vein problems, to take frequent walking breaks while on trips. If traveling by car, simply stop every hour or so and take a brief, brisk walk. If traveling by plane, walk the aisles when the pilot allows you to release your seatbelt.

While traveling in a car or on a plane, I recommend doing toe raises and other leg exercises to keep your calf muscle pump working and the blood moving through your deep veins. When waiting in terminals for flights, elevate your legs. Wearing graduated elastic compression hose during long trips is also helpful in preventing this condition.

Jump through the hoops!

Medical insurance preauthorization for vein treatments can be frustrating. Before preauthorizing reimbursement for the surgical treatment of varicose veins, your insurance company may require that you first try conservative medical measures, such as compression hose, leg elevation, and pain medication. At the risk of offending the medical insurance industry, I'm going take a moment to vent my frustration with this approach.

In my opinion, the logic for trying conservative measures before undergoing treatment procedures seems flawed. These measures may provide temporary relief from symptoms and slow the progression of disease, but they don't address the underlying issues. In most cases, the vein disease will gradually progress in severity, and your risks of blood clots and other complications will increase accordingly.

If this is true, you might be wondering why insurance companies insist that conservative measures first be tried? One of their arguments might be that patients who gain relief from conservative measures are better off because they are able to avoid more invasive procedures. But that line of reasoning is illogical and shortsighted.

Current state-of-the-art vein treatment procedures are substantially more beneficial than conservative treatment measures. And interestingly, the patients who are most likely to benefit from conservative measures are also the most likely to benefit from treatment procedures.

Conservative measures as a long-term solution yield limited benefits. For example, suppose that you experience some relief of symptoms from the use of compression hose. In order for this benefit to continue, you will have to wear compression hose constantly and indefinitely. That's like a lifetime jail sentence! You probably won't do it.

And when you stop wearing the hose, the benefits will cease. At that point you'll either have to live with the debilitating effects of vein disease or undergo surgery. By this time, you may need more extensive surgery because the disease will have progressed.

"A gentleman has no business to concern himself about the legs of a lady."

Abigail Smith in 1764 to her fiancé, future U. S. president John Adams.

I'm a businessman as well as a doctor, so I don't condemn the insurance companies for wanting to reduce costs by avoiding or delaying treatment. But in my opinion, and in the judgment of many of my colleagues, the medical wisdom of this approach is highly questionable. The net effect of these conservative treatment policies, which are not supported by medical studies, is to needlessly delay definitive treatment, which can discourage patients and expose them to unnecessary risks. Ultimately, both patients and insurance companies can incur higher costs.

However, since most insurance companies still require conservative treatment trials, in our practice we will gladly comply with this policy. Upon completion of the trials, we will work with the insurance companies to preauthorize definitive treatment.

No Harm in Asking

Frequently Asked Questions about Vein Disease

OVER THE YEARS MY PATIENTS AND PEOPLE WHO'VE ATTENDED MY SPEAK-
ing engagements have asked lots of interesting questions about
how varicose and spider veins are affected by pregnancy, diet,
weight, sunlight, and even high-heeled shoes. You may have some
of these same questions, so in this chapter I'll answer a few.

Will crossing my legs give me spider veins and varicose veins?

This appears to be an "old wives' tale." There's no medical evidence
that intermittent crossing of the legs causes vein problems. However, sitting in any position for prolonged periods does somewhat
increase your risks.

Do high-heeled shoes cause vein disease?

Although high-heeled shoes can look terrific, they do exacerbate
vein problems because they keep your calf muscles in a contracted,

abnormal position. Calf muscles need to regularly stretch and contract through their full range of motion to maintain their optimal blood-pumping efficiency.

In my opinion, high heels are okay for brief social occasions, but not for prolonged wear. I've treated women who wear them eight to ten hours a day at work, and I would discourage that. Orthopedists and podiatrists who treat foot and ankle conditions have their own set of concerns about how high-heeled shoes affect the bones, ligaments, and tendons in the feet and lower legs.

Does smoking contribute to vein disease?

Smoking and the use of nicotine products are weak risk factors for developing chronic venous insufficiency (CVI). However, it's well established that smoking impairs circulation and can cause coronary disease, heart attacks, strokes, atherosclerosis (hardening of the arteries), and cancer. If you smoke, I strongly encourage you to stop.

In addition to the above problems, smoking can cause peripheral arterial disease (PAD), also known as peripheral vascular disease (PVD). PAD has similar symptoms to CVI—leg pains, skin problems, and poor wound healing—but the two conditions are actually very different.

PAD occurs when insufficient blood flows *into* the legs and feet due to a blockage in the *arteries*. CVI, on the other hand, occurs when insufficient blood flows *out of* the legs and feet though the *veins*. In advanced stages, PAD can cause gangrene that may necessitate amputation. On the other hand, CVI very rarely requires such drastic treatment measures.

If you have leg pains or any of the other symptoms mentioned above, consult a physician right away. If you have a family history of PAD, tell your vein practitioner so this can be taken into account during your evaluation.

If I'm overweight, am I more likely to get vein disease?

Thin people are not immune from varicose and spider veins, but being overweight or obese does elevate your risk. You will usually obtain better treatment results and reduce your chance of recurrence of disease if you shed some of those excess pounds. Nevertheless, I typically won't delay treatments to allow patients to lose weight unless I'm confident of their commitment to follow through.

Does sunlight cause vein disease?

It is unlikely that exposure to ultraviolet (UV) light—either directly from the sun or from artificial tanning lights—increases the risk of leg-vein disease. However, UV light is definitely a risk factor for facial spider veins and vascular blushing (*rosacea*). We do ask patients to avoid exposure to the sun for two to four weeks after leg-vein treatment sessions.

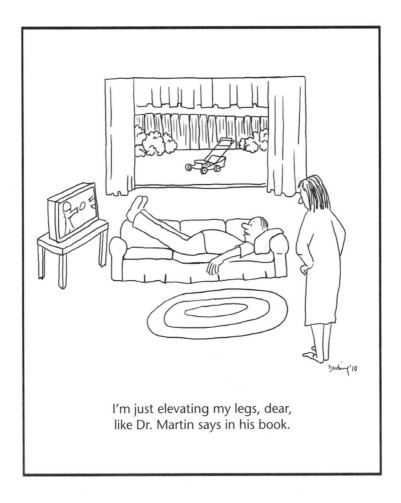

I'm just elevating my legs, dear,
like Dr. Martin says in his book.

Does strenuous exercise increase my risk of getting spider and varicose veins?

Any strenuous exercise, such as weightlifting, that significantly increases the pressure in your abdomen, upper thighs, and groin area could potentially increase your risk of vein problems. The concern arises when pressure on your abdominal area is translated into pressure against your inferior vena cava, which is the main vein that drains blood from the lower half of your body. Pressure on this vein can increase the pressure on other leg veins.

However, because exercise is so vital for good health, I don't advocate eliminating these types of activities. Physical activity exercises and develops the calf-muscle pump, which in turn helps to avoid leg-vein problems. If you have leg-vein problems, you might benefit from wearing compression hose or socks while you are exercising.

What other types of pressure on my abdomen can cause vein problems?

Pregnancy is one of the major risk factors, as we will soon discuss. Also, chronic constipation and tight-fitting jeans and other clothing can cause problems. If you have constipation concerns, I recommend drinking eight to ten glasses of water a day; eating more fruits, vegetables, and whole grains; and adding one or two doses of fiber supplements to your daily diet.

How does pregnancy affect my vein health?

Susceptibility to leg-vein disease and blood clots increases substantially during pregnancy and for up to six months after delivery for the following three reasons:

1. As the fetus in the womb enlarges, it applies increased pressure against the inferior vena cava, the main vein that drains blood from the lower half of the body. In certain body positions, the fetus can practically block the flow of blood. Obstruction of this large vein can dramatically increase vein pressure in the lower body and legs.

2. The volume of blood during pregnancy increases by as much as 50 percent, putting additional stress on leg veins.

3. Pregnancy causes a dramatic spike in the amounts of estrogen, progesterone, and other hormones in the woman's body. In fact, the levels of some hormones during pregnancy increase several millionfold! This causes the smooth muscle of the veins to relax, increasing both their storage capacity and their propensity to dilate. This in turn increases the risk of varicose and spider veins.

The third trimester is the worst time for stress on the legs. Pain, swelling, and other symptoms will often subside or completely resolve in the weeks after delivery, so invasive treatment of spider veins and varicose veins may be avoided unless the problems persist.

If you have leg-vein problems and become pregnant, I encourage you to wear compression hose during your pregnancy and for two weeks after delivery. They can limit the risk of blood clots, slow the progression of vein disease, and provide substantial relief from leg swelling and discomfort. I realize hose can be a nuisance and a discomfort, but the health benefits of wearing them are substantial.

I typically do not offer any treatment that is invasive or requires medication during pregnancy or until after breast-feeding is completed, unless severe pain or disability demands an accelerated schedule. Although the medications used in vein treatments are not known to be harmful to mother or child, they can get into the breast milk. Prudence dictates an abundance of caution.

When vein procedures are advisable before the baby is weaned, I encourage the mother to save some breast milk and freeze it prior to treatment. During treatment and for one day following, she can thaw the milk and feed it to the baby. During this time, the mother will continue to pump her breasts and discard the milk ("pump and dump") as the medications clear out of her body. Normal breast-feeding can be resumed 48 hours after the venous treatment.

What about anti-inflammatory pain medications for relief of leg-disease discomfort?

For temporary relief of leg pain and discomfort, I often recommend anti-inflammatory pain medications that can be purchased off the shelf. There are many available, but the most popular and my favorite is ibuprofen (brand names: Motrin or Advil). I advise adults to take two to four 200mg tablets three times a day, or no more frequently than every six hours.

Naproxen (brand name: Aleve) is a good alternative. It is a little less potent than ibuprofen, but longer lasting. One 220mg tablet twice a day (every 12 hours) is usually sufficient.

All anti-inflammatory pain medications increase stomach acid output. For this reason, patients who are prone to stomach upset, ulcers, gastritis, or heartburn (reflux) problems might want to either avoid them or combine them with medications that reduce stomach acid output, such as Pepcid, Zantac, Prilosec, or Tagamet. Other pain medications with anti-inflammatory properties are available by prescription.

Acetaminophen (brand name: Tylenol) is another mild pain medication that is available off the shelf. Although it does not have anti-inflammatory properties, it does have the advantage of not increasing stomach acid output or kidney toxicity. For this reason, it is a good option for patients with kidney complications or stomach concerns. Caution: Do not take this medication with or following alcohol use due to liver toxicity concerns.

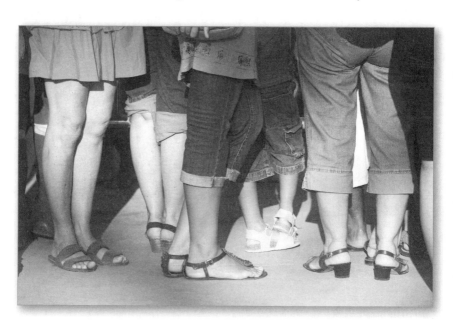

Are any natural remedies effective in the treatment of varicose and spider veins?

A number of natural supplements and herbal products have been recommended and marketed for the prevention and treatment of vein disease. Some of the most common are described below:

- Horse chestnut seed extract, taken in 300-mg doses three times per day, is popular in Europe as a conservative treatment for leg-vein disease. Medical studies seem to indicate that this herbal product relieves some discomfort and swelling.[5]

  I sometimes recommend this homeopathic remedy to patients who for philosophical or other reasons wish to delay or avoid other types of medical treatments. Many have reported good results. However, benefits are only derived while the herb is being used. Symptoms return immediately after treatment is stopped.

- Some natural medications, referred to as venotonic agents and rutosides (sometimes our British colleagues call them phlebotonic agents), increase the contraction capabilities, or tone, of veins, and thus can provide temporary relief from the pain and swelling associated with vein disease. They are more popular and available in Europe than in the United States.

- Vitamin K helps the liver manufacture blood-clotting protein factors, which are important for good health. However, to my knowledge, there's no evidence it is beneficial for the treatment or prevention of varicose veins or spider veins.

- According to some, vitamin C strengthens the walls of veins, but I'm unaware of any reliable research that supports this claim.

- Blueberries, bilberries, gingko, wheat grass, vitamin E, vitamin B-6, grape seed extract (*resveratrol*), raspberries, cherry juice, and a wide variety of antioxidant bioflavonoids (citrus fruits, tea, red wine, dark chocolate) have all been mentioned in connection with vein health. However, I'm unaware that any of the above has been proven to be beneficial.

- Some advertisements I have read claim that witch hazel will decrease varicose vein discomfort by tightening the skin and reducing inflammation, but I have not seen this medically substantiated. Older patients have told me that using witch hazel helps relieve their symptoms.

Can spider veins or varicose veins cause bleeding emergencies?

Bleeding from ruptured or injured veins is rather uncommon; I only see a few cases a year. It's remarkable how infrequently this condition occurs, actually, because the skin overlying varicose and spider veins is often extraordinarily thin, and the pressures within varicose veins are quite high.

If you do happen to experience this type of hemorrhage, the bleeding can be brisk. But don't panic. Lie down and elevate the leg that is bleeding to reduce the pressure. Next, hold direct pressure over the bleeding site using tissue paper, gauze, a clean piece of cloth, or even the tip of your finger. In most cases, bleeding will stop within seven minutes. I advise holding firm pressure over the site for fifteen to thirty minutes.

If bleeding persists for more than thirty minutes, proceed immediately—by ambulance, if necessary—to a physician's office or to the emergency room of a hospital. As soon as possible after the emergency has passed, see a vein specialist. Bleeding at hemorrhage sites tends to recur. Definitive treatment of the abnormal veins should eliminate the risk of recurrent bleeding.

---

5. "Horse Chestnut Seed Extract," in *Herbal Medicine Expanded commission E Monographs*, eds. M. Blumenthal, A. Goldberg, and J. Brinckman. (Newton, MA: Lippencott Williams & Wilkens, 2000), 201-204.

Finding the Right Doctor

When and How to Seek Professional Help

I STRONGLY RECOMMEND SEEING A VEIN SPECIALIST FOR AN ASSESSMENT if you have or have had any of the following conditions:

- Blood-clot complications or hemorrhaging of your leg veins
- Vein-related wounds (*venous stasis ulcerations*)
- Varicose veins
- Symptoms of chronic venous insufficiency (CVI), such as discomfort, tiredness, pain, or swelling in your legs and feet

Vein specialists have the training and the technology, including color-flow duplex ultrasound capabilities, to make accurate assessments and prescribe the most effective treatments. Primary care physicians or other medical practitioners who do not specialize in the treatment of vein disease typically don't.

Better now than later

Leg-vein disease is progressive. Left unattended, a few spider veins are likely to progress into many spider veins or, even worse, varicose veins. If you have any of the conditions mentioned above, even if your symptoms are mild and non-debilitating, you should see a vein specialist for an assessment and possible treatment.

Early intervention can slow the progression of disease and prevent future problems. It can also reduce the number of treatments required. Postponing treatments exposes you to increased risk of blood-clot complications, including superficial phlebitis and the more serious deep vein thrombosis (DVT).

In years past, people tended to postpone leg-vein treatments as long as possible. There was some logic to that because the older procedures were only marginally effective and often had to be repeated every few years.

But times have changed. Modern techniques treat the root causes of vein disease, so the results are comprehensive and durable. I tell patients that my goal is to make their legs look and feel better, not just for the next five years, but for the rest of their lives.

Chronic venous insufficiency problems that at first seem minor can eventually cause physical limitations and disability, even in young people. I've cared for CVI patients in their twenties and thirties who have been declared medically disabled and are receiving government benefits.

Most of my patients are pleasantly surprised to see how these treatments can relieve discomfort, eliminate disabilities, and give them more stamina on their feet. Often those who were disabled return to work and resume exercising.

Quality of life is a health issue.

Many of my spider vein patients, especially women, seek treatment primarily for cosmetic reasons. Some are so embarrassed about how they look in shorts, skirts, and sandals that they will wear heavier clothing to hide their legs, even in sweltering heat.

In my opinion, unsightly legs and feet that curtail lifestyles and damage self-esteem are substantial health issues. If you have aesthetic concerns, there's no advantage in postponing treatment. To gain maximum lifetime health benefits, sooner and younger is better.

Treatments for varicose and spider veins typically provide both cosmetic and medical benefits. I often joke with my patients, "If this procedure doesn't improve your medical problems or symptoms, at least you'll have better looking legs!" Most of the time, they get both.

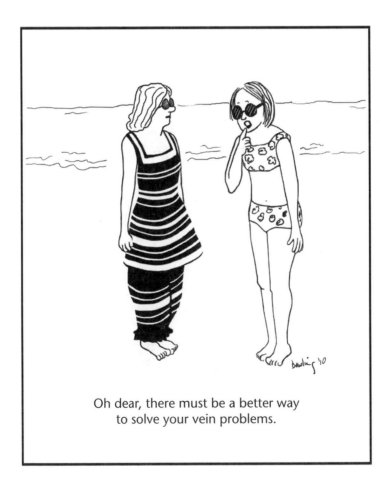

Oh dear, there must be a better way
to solve your vein problems.

What type of physician is best?

Many different physicians in a variety of specialties are now treating vein diseases. I have friends and respected colleagues in the fields of family medicine, internal medicine, dermatology, emergency medicine, obstetrics and gynecology, and interventional radiology who are doing outstanding work with venous insufficiency problems. The myriad of specialists offering vein treatments makes finding the right doctor more challenging.

At the annual meeting of the American College of Phlebology in 2007, I admit to being both surprised and disappointed that only about 30 percent of the attending physicians were surgeons. Board-certified surgeons, it seems to me, are ideally positioned to treat vein diseases. Their knowledge of leg-vein anatomy and state-of-the-art surgical techniques, bolstered by any experiences they may have had with the older leg-vein treatment methods, should give them an advantage over physicians in non-surgical specialties.

Surgeons also are best qualified through knowledge and training to handle complications that might arise during the treatment of varicose veins and other serious issues. A non-surgeon, on the other hand, may have to abort treatment and refer the patient to another specialist.

When I use the term "board-certified surgeons," I'm primarily referring to vascular surgeons, general surgeons, cardiothoracic surgeons, and plastic surgeons. Vascular surgeons, in particular, have traditionally focused on vein medicine because they specialize in treating diseases of the blood vessels.

It's worth noting, however, that although vascular surgeons treat both arteries and veins, they devote the great majority of their attention to diseases of the arteries. Frankly, vein diseases are the stepchild of the vascular surgery specialty. Even most vascular surgery medical textbooks relegate the vein chapters to the back of the book.

I don't mean to be critical. The emphasis vascular surgeons place on arterial disease is probably justified. Diseases of the arteries generally are more likely to develop into problems that threaten overall health and life.

But here's the irony. Even though diseases of the arteries get more attention from vascular surgeons, diseases of the veins are more common in patients. And the patients who suffer from them are often strongly motivated to seek treatment.

Perhaps in future years more surgeons, vascular surgeons in particular, will decide to specialize in vein medicine. In fact, at a recent American Venous Forum national meeting, vascular surgeons were the dominant specialty in attendance. Many of their discussions revolved around phrases such as "catching up" or "taking back." I would agree.

Finding the right doctor for you

When seeking professional medical care, ask other people who suffer from conditions similar to yours for their advice. Find out which doctors they respect and why.

It's always wise to ask your primary care physician for recommendations and guidance. Be mindful, however, that many primary care physicians are not fully aware of the new state-of-the-art treatments available for vein diseases. Medical information is expanding at an exponential rate, and every physician has difficulty keeping abreast of new developments.

In my opinion, modern treatment methods for varicose and spider veins are at least twenty times better today than they were only ten years ago. However, some doctors still have less-than-favorable perceptions of vein medicine based on outdated information. So don't be surprised if your general practitioner is not as knowledgeable or encouraging as you would like. As you look for a qualified vein specialist, you may find yourself largely on your own.

Some words of caution

As the advances in vein medicine become more widely known and appreciated, quite a number of doctors are attempting to add vein treatments as one aspect of their practices. Some companies are even offering weekend workshops to teach doctors how to increase revenues by treating varicose and spider veins with the new laser or radiofrequency technologies.

If I were a patient, this type of "dabbling" would concern me. Doctors who make a half-hearted commitment to vein medicine could potentially do a disservice to their patients and to the profession.

To be proficient, I think a physician needs to dedicate a minimum of two days per week to treating vein problems. Optimally, I recommend looking for a vein practitioner who has been treating vein problems on a full-time basis for at least two years.

Some physicians have the impression that vein diseases are relatively easy to treat, but that's far from the truth. Vein medicine is extremely challenging. It takes time and effort to learn the new techniques, especially for the treatment of varicose veins. There's a definite learning curve. Physicians who practice vein medicine on a part-time basis will have difficulty gaining the experience necessary for proficiency.

Before you select a doctor, find out how many major varicose vein disease cases he or she has treated. Experience is important. Fewer than 150 to 200 cases is cause for concern. I've performed more than 6,000 endovenous ablation procedures and tens of thousands of spider vein treatments, and I'm still learning.

By the way, when I suggest choosing a physician who has performed at least 150 vein operations, I realize I'm presenting a "Catch 22." Don't ask me who my first 150 patients were!

Venous professional organizations

Phlebology is the art and science of assessing and treating vein disease. In 2007, it was approved by the American Medical Association for inclusion in its list of self-designated medical specialties. It is recognized as a medical specialty by a number of state medical boards. The American College of Phlebology has expanded its efforts to seek certificate recognition by the American Board of Medical Specialties.

In recent years, several organizations have been organized to foster the development of this emerging field of medicine and oversee its professional quality. I've listed some in appendix B. Their websites may be a useful resource to you as you search for a vein specialist. Many of the more experienced and better trained vein practitioners belong to one or more of these organizations.

Getting to Know You

What to Expect of Your Initial Consultation

LET'S SUPPOSE THAT YOU'VE DECIDED TO SEE A VEIN SPECIALIST. PERHAPS you've even identified one or more physicians you'd like to visit. In this chapter we'll talk about what you can expect when you go in for your initial consultation and evaluation.

Your initial consultation

Your initial session with your doctor should last about thirty to sixty minutes. At the conclusion of the exam, your physician should be able to recommend treatment options, if appropriate.

Varicose veins and spider veins are easily recognizable from their distinct visual patterns, so I can often assess the condition of a patient's legs from their appearance. But I always rely on ultrasound techniques to confirm my diagnosis and guide treatment. The patient's symptoms are the most important factor to consider when formulating a treatment recommendation.

In years past, many venous x-ray exams were performed by radiologists using venogram diagnostic techniques. An IV was placed in the patient's foot and a dye was injected into the leg veins. In addition to being somewhat expensive, invasive, and painful, this exam could aggravate kidney disease. That's why it is seldom used today.

Color-flow venous duplex ultrasound has emerged as the new gold standard for detecting and treating chronic venous insufficiency. It is comfortable, safe, and noninvasive. It's considered so safe, in fact, that physicians routinely use it to examine a fetus during pregnancy.

How ultrasound works

Ultrasound equipment transmits and receives ultrahigh-frequency sound waves (too high to be heard with the human ear) through a sensor that is placed in contact with the legs. Transmission gel applied to the legs facilitates passage of the ultrasound waves between the sensor's transmitter and receiver.

With this state-of-the-art technology, a qualified examiner can easily and accurately determine the diameter and location of veins and identify valve leakages. The color-flow feature utilizes the Doppler effect[6] to determine and depict the movement of blood.

During an examination, I apply a bit of pressure to the patient's calf muscle to force blood up the leg veins. The ultrasound monitor displays this flow in blue. When I release the pressure, there should be no downward movement of blood if the vein valves are functioning properly, so the image of the vein will remain black. However, if the valves in the vein are insufficient, blood falling back down the leg will show up in red on the screen.

Ultrasound takes the guesswork out of diagnosing vein disease. Before the advent of this remarkable technology, physicians would sometimes strip the wrong veins or fail to treat veins that were defective. That's a major reason why the older methods of treating vein disease were less than satisfactory. Physicians, especially surgeons with experience in vein stripping and the older treatment methods, are uniquely qualified to recognize unusual anatomy variations or complications resulting from procedures that are now considered obsolete.

Experience and training matter

Although ultrasound is an extraordinary tool, its effectiveness depends largely on the knowledge and experience of the examiner. Most ultrasounds are performed by ultrasound technologists, who are radiology technologists with additional training. They are excellent at what they do, but in my opinion leg venous ultrasound exams should be performed by a registered vascular technologist (RVT). RVT is a certification offered by the American Registry of Diagnostic Medical Sonographers (ARDMS).

I wish to insert a word of caution here. Although RVTs are well-trained professionals, they primarily perform ultrasound exams to assess deep vein thrombosis (DVT) and blood-clot problems. During these exams, patients are usually in a supine rather than a standing position, and that's perfectly appropriate.

However, to detect venous reflux problems, the patient should be in a standing position. This allows the examiner to perform leg compression maneuvers, especially of the calf and thigh muscles, and use the color-flow duplex feature of the ultrasound to determine which valves are leaking.

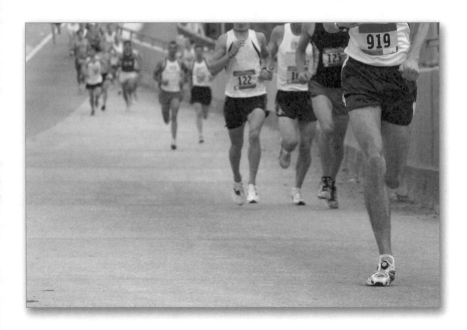

Not infrequently patients come to me who have had ultrasound examinations performed at a hospital or in their physician's office. Although these exams usually detect any active blood-clot complications, they provide little or no useful information for addressing such CVI issues as long-term pain, swelling, or varicose veins.

That's why I believe that physicians who specialize in the treatment of vein disease should take the time and effort to obtain RVT qualification. To deliver the best quality care, they should perform their own ultrasound examinations and use ultrasound to guide them in treatment.

I don't mean to be critical of ultrasound technicians. Most are highly qualified and excellent at detecting blood-clot complications and deep vein thrombosis. But they often don't have the necessary training to assess chronic venous insufficiency and varicose vein disease. However, I'm encouraged to see that many more technicians are learning to do venous reflux examinations correctly.

Questions to ask during the initial consultation

During your initial consultation, gather all of the necessary information before you commit to treatment. Below are some suggested questions to ask:

- What are my treatment options?
- What is the one best option for me, and why?
- What specific experience do you have with this particular technique?
- What are the risks of having the procedure?
- What are the risks of *not* having the procedure?
- What can I expect the recovery to be like, and what is the timeline?
- What are the typical side effects?
- What type of follow-up plan and schedule will I have?

6. *The Doppler effect* (or *Doppler shift*), named after Austrian physicist Christian Doppler, who proposed it in 1842, is the change in frequency of a wave for an observer moving relative to the source of the wave. This effect is commonly heard when a vehicle sounding a siren or horn approaches, passes, and recedes from an observer. The received frequency gets higher (compared to the emitted frequency) during the approach; it is identical at the instant of passing by; and it grows lower during the recession.

Section Two

Spider Veins: Diagnoses, Causes, and Treatments

CHAPTER EIGHT

Up Comes the Spider

How Those Spider Veins Got on Your Legs

SPIDER VEINS ARE THE TINY VEINS—USUALLY PURPLE, RED, OR BLUE IN color—that sometimes appear in the superficial layer of the skin (the *epidermis*). As the name implies, the individual veins emanating out from a central cluster can resemble the legs of a spider.

Spider veins eventually present themselves in approximately 70 percent of adult females, and a smaller percentage of males. Many people view them as simply a cosmetic problem. But in about two-thirds of the cases, spider veins are responsible for some degree of medical discomfort or disability.

The most common symptoms associated with spider veins are pain, burning, heaviness, itching, stinging, swelling, restlessness, and fatigue in the legs. People with spider veins also run a somewhat higher risk of suffering from superficial thrombophlebitis[7] in their legs over the course of their lifetime. Therefore, the majority of spider vein treatments address both medical and cosmetic concerns.

Many patients seek spider vein treatments strictly for cosmetic reasons. After treatment, however, they are often amazed at how much lighter, fresher, and more energetic their legs feel. They are surprised to learn that the chronic heaviness and fatigue in their legs that they had unconsciously lived with for so long was in fact abnormal, and not a necessary result of the aging process.

Bobby Smith's Story

Bobby Smith, age 73, is retired from a forty-year career in a pulp mill.

In the early days when I worked at the pulp mill, they didn't have all the safety regulations they have today. Sometimes my legs would get burned by the chlorine and caustic soda chemicals we used. On top of that, I had a bad case of varicose and spider veins, so my legs were in really bad shape.

When I was in my late forties or early fifties, I was suffering so much from varicose veins in my left leg that I went in for one of those vein-stripping procedures. That really did me more harm than good. My left leg swelled up so bad I couldn't see my ankle. It never did get back to normal size. So I lived with that bad leg for years.

Not long ago, my brother went to see Dr. Martin to have his spider veins treated. He kept telling me how much better it made his legs feel, so I asked my regular doctor for his opinion. He said he didn't know much about the new treatments for vein disease, but that he would be interested to see if they could help me.

Dr. Martin told me that my varicose veins were some of the worst he had ever seen. I had three large varicose veins that had disintegrated. He treated my left leg first, and then my right leg. I could tell the difference almost immediately. They didn't feel tired and heavy like they used to. I've been back for several treatments since then, and my legs keep getting better.

On my next visit to my regular doctor, he said, "My goodness! What did you do to your legs?" He was so impressed with how good they looked! I don't have any more swelling in my legs. I can walk without pain, and I can even ride a bicycle. My wife has been in to see Dr. Martin, too, and her legs look and feel a lot better. I've referred a lot of people to him.

What causes spider veins?

Spider veins, like all chronic venous insufficiency problems, are caused by leaky valves in the veins of the leg that allow blood to fall sluggishly downward, instead of briskly flowing upward as it should. During prolonged periods of sitting or standing, the pooling blood accumulates under increasing pressure below the leaky valves, causing the vein to become inflamed and dilated.

But spider veins themselves are just the tip of the iceberg. Two even bigger culprits lurk beneath the skin's surface. One of these villains goes by the name of "incompetent reticular vein."

That's the standard medical term for a larger vein that lies just below the surface of the skin. I and many of my colleagues refer to them simply as *feeding green veins*. That's because in fair-skinned patients they're greenish-blue in color, and they "feed" blood at excessive pressures into clusters of spider veins. Other physicians refer to them as *blue-green veins* or *root veins*. (Every villain must have a few aliases!)

The other culprit is the *incompetent perforator vein*. Perforator veins are short connecting blood vessels that carry blood from your superficial vein system inward to your deep vein system. Your deep veins then transport the blood briskly up your legs and back to your heart and lungs for replenishment with oxygen.

A valve within each perforator vein allows blood to flow in only one direction: from the superficial veins to the deep veins. But if this valve becomes defective and leaks (i.e., the perforator vein becomes incompetent), blood begins to flow backwards from the deep veins to the superficial veins.

Blood flowing in the wrong direction through feeding green veins and incompetent perforator veins creates pressure on the superficial vein system immediately beneath the skin. According to one theory, spider veins form at the surface of the skin when the body attempts to alleviate this pressure.

Feeding green veins are enemy #1!

The best way—in fact, the only effective way—to get rid of spider veins is to close the feeding green veins. It's even more important to treat the feeding green veins than it is to treat the spider veins themselves.

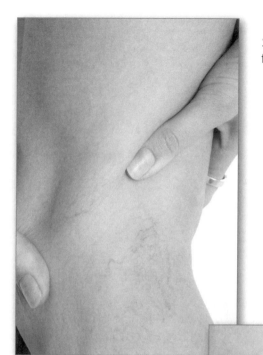

Spider veins with
feeding green veins

Spider veins

But a decade ago, most physicians didn't know this. If they had, they couldn't have done much about it anyway, because the medical techniques at that point simply weren't up to the task.

Hypertonic saline injections and spider vein laser therapies are just "surface treatments" that ignore the underlying disease process. So, until fairly recently we physicians treated spider veins while ignoring the underlying feeding green veins. No wonder the results were limited and transitory! To get back to our gardening analogy, we were cutting off the weeds and leaving the roots behind.

Fortunately, that all has changed. As we're about to discuss, we now have excellent methods for treating feeding green veins. And to add to the good news, we are able to automatically close incompetent perforator veins by simply treating the adjoining feeding green veins. However, very large incompetent perforator veins may need additional treatment, as we will discuss in chapter 15.

Spiders on your legs

An incompetent lateral venous system in a female is the most common pattern of abnormal veins that produces spider veins. It has a strong genetic tendency that is increased by pregnancy and physical activity. Note in the top photograph on page 56 that the pattern of feeding green veins is distinct and easily recognizable. The largest feeding green veins in females are on the outside, or lateral aspect, of the thighs, knees, and calves. Smaller branches occur throughout the legs.

The vein of Albanese is the largest feeding green vein. As shown in this photograph, it runs along the outside or lateral aspect of the thigh. In fair-skinned patients, it can often be seen with the naked eye.

There's usually an area in the center of the outside of the thigh, knee, and calf where the skin is clear of spider veins. But beyond this clear central area, spider veins will splay and branch out on the skin's surface from the underlying feeding green veins. These clusters often resemble a sunburst arch, as you can see in the bottom photograph.

Men also have feeding green veins, but they develop in a more random pattern throughout the legs. Nevertheless, the treatment methods for men and women may be similar.

Getting rid of incompetent veins

We'll get more into how we treat abnormal veins in the succeeding chapters. But at this point it's sufficient to say that we "destroy" them. That may sound harsh, but spider veins, feeding green veins, and incompetent perforator veins are pathological. In other words, they aren't supposed to be there.

"Hold on!" my patients often say. "Don't I need all my veins? Won't eliminating these abnormal veins harm the blood circulation in my legs?"

That's a reasonable question. I've even been asked it by a number of primary care physicians. However, nothing could be further from the truth. The confusion may arise because there is very little redundancy in your artery system, and it is critical to preserve as many of the arteries in your legs as possible. However, there is a lot of redundancy in the vein system, and you have many more veins in your legs than necessary for good health.

Blood flows through abnormal, incompetent veins sluggishly and under abnormally high pressure. This is an unhealthy, abnormal state. Not only can this condition produce pain, swelling, and the various other symptoms we have discussed, it also increases the risk of phlebitis and blood clots.

When we destroy abnormal veins, the flow of blood is redirected through tributary veins to nearby healthy veins that have properly functioning valves. Unlike the sluggish, high-pressure flow of blood through abnormal veins, the blood through healthy veins flows briskly and efficiently upward through your legs back toward your heart, as God intended when He designed your body.

You actually have many more veins in your legs than you need. Getting rid of defective ones improves circulation and health. This is why you will often experience relief of discomfort and other symptoms after treatment, and your legs will feel fresher and lighter.

---

7. See appendix A for a glossary of medical terms.

The Medical Revolution

Spider Vein Treatments, Past and Present

UNTIL QUITE RECENTLY, THE GREAT MAJORITY OF PHYSICIANS TREATED SPIder veins by injecting them with hypertonic saline medication. This agent is essentially pharmacy-grade sodium chloride (salt water) whose concentration (11.7%) exceeds that of the body's blood and tissues.[8]

Although these injections close the spider veins, the results are limited and short-lived. That's because this procedure only treats the spider veins on the skin's surface and is largely ineffective in closing the underlying feeding green veins, which are the root cause of spider veins.

In addition, hypertonic saline injections can produce substantial pain and burning, lingering muscle cramps, and other undesirable side effects. You should be aware that some medical practitioners still use this procedure to treat spider veins, even though it is considered by many to be obsolete.

The new "gold standard"

In the past decade a new "gold standard" treatment for spider veins has emerged. Sclerotherapy injection of foam medication into feeding green veins produces results manyfold better than hypertonic saline injections into spider veins.

Sclerotherapy is a minimally invasive procedure for the treatment of spider veins that is performed in an office setting on an outpatient basis. The term "sclerotherapy" comes from the Greek word "sclero," which means "to harden." With sclerotherapy, the physician destroys (ablates) the abnormal veins by injecting medication directly into them using very small needles.

There are several different sclerotherapy medicines. Each agent has advantages and disadvantages, but all are designed to chemically injure the inside walls of the defective veins. The resulting inflammation causes the vein to collapse and close, cutting off all blood flow through it. Ultimately, it will convert to scar tissue, disintegrate (involute), and be absorbed by the body.

Some of the smaller veins disappear instantly. Medium-sized spider veins typically take two to six weeks to vanish. Some of the larger spider veins and feeding green veins may take two to four months to completely fade from sight.

If you desire treatment for spider veins, I encourage you to find a practitioner who is experienced in this new sclerotherapy technique. There is no "second best" in the medical world today. All other treatment methods are substantial compromises. With this state-of-the-art treatment procedure, you should experience symptom relief for many years. I'll provide more details about this procedure in the next chapter.

The new medications

Since new and better medications are a significant reason for the dramatic improvement in sclerotherapy treatment results, I'll give you some basic information about them so you can be sure you are receiving state-of-the-art treatment. It is perfectly appropriate to ask your physician which medications he or she plans to use.

The most prevalent medication used today by well-trained vein specialists in the United States is the chemical detergent agent sodium tetradecyl sulfate. It is manufactured by Bioniche Pharma USA under the trade name Sotradecol.

Sotradecol comes in a liquid version that most practitioners use for treating smaller spider veins. Some also inject larger spider veins and feeding green veins with the liquid form of the medication.

However, because the flow of blood in larger veins tends to flush liquid medicines away before they can sufficiently damage the vein walls, I prefer to convert the liquid to foam for treating larger abnormal veins. The foam version of the medicine is more technically challenging to administer, but it results in better clearing with less risk of staining of the skin.

The medical use of chemical detergent agents for sclerotherapy dates back to the late 1930s and early 1940s, but for some reason these medications fell out of vogue for decades. Perhaps World War II was a distracting factor. Happily, they were "rediscovered" in the late 1990s and have since enjoyed a popular, worldwide resurgence.

The advantages of newer sclerotherapy agents

Sotradecol has several advantages over hypertonic saline and other similar medicines. One major advantage is its chemical structure, which allows it to be converted into foam (suds). In our office, we convert the liquid to foam at the moment of treatment by mixing (agitating) it with air or gas using a standardized protocol.

The foam version of the medication is dramatically more effective and potent than the liquid version, especially for the larger-caliber (larger-diameter) feeding green veins. With micro-bubbles and a consistency somewhat like diluted shaving cream, it's thicker and stickier than its liquid counterpart. The foam medicine adheres to the inside walls (endothelium) of the larger veins longer and does a beautiful job of drying up the feeding green veins. It can also be used on smaller varicose veins.

I sometimes inject diluted foam medicine directly into the spider veins. This is technically more difficult, and I only know of a few practitioners who attempt it. Most use the liquid agent for the spider veins and reserve the foam agent for the underlying feeding green veins.

No additional treatment is needed for the incompetent perforator veins in the setting of spider vein therapy. Foam injected into abnormal feeding green veins naturally flows into the adjoining small perforator veins, closing and sealing them. The process just described has been the real key to dramatic improvements in the treatment of spider veins. Further therapy may be needed for large perforator veins in the context of varicose vein treatment or severe venous insufficiency.

Alternatives to Sotradecol

Outside the United States, the most popular sclerotherapy agent is Aethoxysklerol, or polidocanol. I think of it as Sotradecol's cousin because it's also a chemical detergent agent with similar properties.

Polidocanol was recently approved for use in the United States by the Federal Drug Administration (FDA) under the brand name Asclera.[9] Because the risk of side effects is slightly less with Asclera than with Sotradecol, and since it is a little more comfortable upon injection, I expect it will enjoy strong popularity in the United States.

In the past, most vein practitioners converted liquid Sotradecol and polidocanol to foam by mixing it with air. But there's a recent trend toward the use of carbon dioxide instead of air, because it is absorbed much faster into the bloodstream. This may improve the safety of treatment. However, Sotradecol mixed with carbon dioxide is less stable (i.e., it tends to return to the liquid form more quickly), which makes it more difficult to use.

Varisolve[10] is a new foam agent that at the time of this writing is undergoing the FDA study process. It is essentially the same medicine as polidocanol, except that it is pre-foamed with a mixture of carbon dioxide and oxygen. Varisolve gases are more rapidly absorbed by the body, and its foam is more stable than foams made from carbon dioxide alone.

Limitations on treatment

Women who are pregnant or breast-feeding should not undergo sclerotherapy. Also, anyone who suffers from heart failure, active infections, uncontrolled diabetes, or other illnesses should postpone treatment until these conditions are resolved.

If you take blood-thinning medications, tell your vein specialist. Although the risks of bleeding problems are minimal with our current medical agents, your doctor may recommend temporarily stopping these medications before starting sclerotherapy. This applies to all blood-thinning medications, including such milder medicines as aspirin and Plavix, and to any anti-inflammatory medications used to combat inflammation or arthritis.

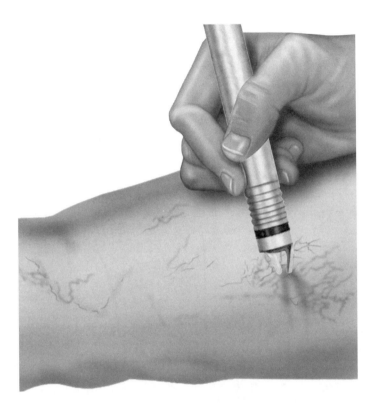

Fig. 9.1 Dornier's SkinPulse 940-nm diode laser being used to ablate leg spider veins. Laser treatments can be successful if they are coupled with treatment of the underlying incompetent feeding green veins.

Laser technology

For the past twenty years or so, lasers have been commonly used to treat spider veins. The word LASER is an acronym for Light Amplification by Stimulated Emission of Radiation. A laser delivers a single wavelength of intense electromagnetic radiation (light energy) directly onto the vein, burning it and causing it to seal. Gradually the damaged vein will wither and be absorbed into the body.

However, unless laser treatments are coupled with state-of-the-art foam sclerotherapy to close the underlying feeding green veins, they provide only temporary improvement at best. Used alone, lasers can actually aggravate spider vein problems over the long term. Like garden weeds that have been cut instead of pulled up by their roots, the spider veins will ultimately return, often worse than before.

The state-of-the-art methods for treating spider veins represent a significant improvement over past methods. In addition to providing excellent relief from current symptoms, they will keep the majority of spider veins from recurring. And perhaps most importantly, they will prevent the development of new spider veins and varicose veins in future years.

Often I tell patients that my goal is for their legs to look and feel better, not only presently, but in five years, twenty years, and to a substantial degree for the rest of their lives. Our new treatment methods make this possible because they allow us to eliminate the worst and largest feeding green veins.

Intense pulse light (IPL) therapy

Several new techniques have emerged in the past few years for treating spider veins, in addition to chemical agent sclerotherapy and lasers. Intense pulse light (IPL) therapy and thermocoagulation (also called electrodessication) are two worth noting.

In contrast to lasers, which pinpoint a single wavelength of light at specific spider veins, IPL therapy applies a broadband of many wavelengths of light to larger areas of skin. The energy absorption from IPL can clear very small spider veins and reduce the size of medium spider veins.

IPL can occasionally be an effective tool for accelerating the clearing of matted spider veins. However, it is not a good primary means of treatment because it does not adequately treat feeding green veins or larger spider veins.

Thermocoagulation

With thermocoagulation, also called ohmic thermolysis, fine needle probes placed in contact with spider veins at the skin's surface deliver electrical energy that destroys spider veins instantly. You will experience a brief pinprick sensation that is mildly discomforting, but there are no open wounds

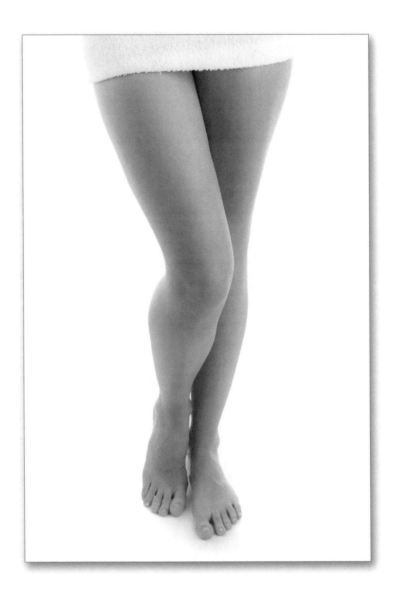

and no need for bandages. Substantial clearing is usually achieved in one to three sessions.

Thermocoagulation is a very safe and effective treatment modality for small spider veins on the legs or face. But like lasers, it treats only the surface of the skin, so, for durable results in the legs, it should be combined with foam sclerotherapy treatment of feeding green veins and larger spider veins. One major advantage it has over lasers, however, is that it can be used on patients with dark skin pigmentation and tans. Veinwave and Vein-Gogh are two companies that offer this technology.

All spider vein treatment methods are "lunchtime procedures." After treatment, you can return immediately to work; virtually no recovery period is needed. I advise long, brisk walks to accelerate healing and lower the risk of blood-clot complications. However, running, weightlifting, or other strenuous exercises should be avoided for at least one week.

A word of warning

Be wary of practitioners who are not vein specialists, but who provide these types of treatments. Unfortunately, some physicians without the proper training seek to augment their income by offering these techniques, but their standard of care is usually less than satisfactory.

In my opinion, leg-vein problems should not be treated unless leg-vein circulation is first assessed, possibly with the aid of ultrasound. Laser, IPL, and thermocoagulation procedures should be performed only in conjunction with foam sclerotherapy of the feeding green veins.

Now that you know a bit about the medications and technologies used in treating spider veins, we will talk in the next chapter about the actual treatment protocol.

---

8. Glycerin, sodium morrhuate, and several other chemical agents that were once commonly used and are still in limited use today also have major drawbacks. Sodium morrhuate, for example, has been linked to severe allergic reactions (anaphylaxis).

9. Manufactured by Chemische Fabreik Kreussler & Co. and available in the United States from BioForm Medical, Inc.

10. Developed by BTG of the United Kingdom

Sclerotherapy Isn't Scary

Spider Vein Treatment Protocol

IF YOU ARE CONTEMPLATING TREATMENT FOR SPIDER VEINS, YOU'LL PROBably feel more comfortable knowing what's involved. The protocol that I and most other experienced vein specialists follow is very straightforward.

After cleaning and sterilizing the surface of your skin, usually with rubbing alcohol, I'll use tiny needles to inject sclerotherapy medication directly into the spider veins on the surface of your skin. Then I'll inject your underlying feeding green veins with a more concentrated foam version of the medication.

After dimming the room lights, I'll place a transilluminating vein light on the skin's surface to help me locate veins. The skin and fat layers glow orange, while the feeding green veins show up as contrasting dark lines.

Sessions generally last about fifteen to thirty minutes, but they can run as long as an hour. I try to work quickly and gently so you'll barely feel the majority of the injections. They will cause about as much discomfort as a modest pinch, although a vein that happens to be close to a sensory nerve branch can be a little more sensitive. Knees, ankles, and feet also tend to be more sensitive because they have more sensory nerves.

Relaxing at the office

If you have "needle phobia"—perhaps because of unpleasant experiences with the larger needles used for shots, IVs, and drawing blood—you needn't be anxious. Sclerotherapy employs a very fine needle, so it's a different ballgame.

It's best to just relax and let the sensations come and go. If there is discomfort, it's only momentary. I attempt to minimize anxiety by carrying on a reassuring conversation, playing music, and telling jokes so ineptly that they're sometimes funny.

In the initial two sessions I usually treat only one leg at a time. This allows me to be thorough without exceeding the maximum recommended dosage for the sclerotherapy medication. In subsequent sessions, because the abnormal veins are fewer and smaller, I can usually treat both legs during the same visit without exceeding the dosage and foam-volume limits of the medication.

In the interest of limiting fees or discomfort, patients sometimes ask me to treat a specific patch of spider veins, or to treat the abnormal veins only from the knee down. But treating only a portion of a leg is not advisable. The excessive overflow pressure from other feeding green veins in neighboring areas will result in poor treatment results over the long term. It's important to treat the entire leg.

Better and better

Your response to sclerotherapy will vary, depending on the severity of your disease, your age, your state of health, and other factors. In our practice, however, we expect about 70 percent clearing of abnormal veins after each treatment session.

Three to six treatments are usually advisable for spider veins, because each treatment builds on the results of the previous one. If you're in your teens or early twenties and have only mild spider veins, you may be satisfied with the results after one or two sessions. If you're older, you will probably need more. Discuss this with your treating physician.

Scheduling follow-up sessions four to eight weeks apart gives your body time to reroute the flow of blood to healthy veins, relieving stress on the vein system. This allows me to more accurately assess which additional veins need to be treated. The time interval also allows for clearing of bruising and inflammation from the prior treatment. If patients are eager to complete a series of treatments, I will sometimes shorten this interval to three weeks, but that's an absolute minimum.

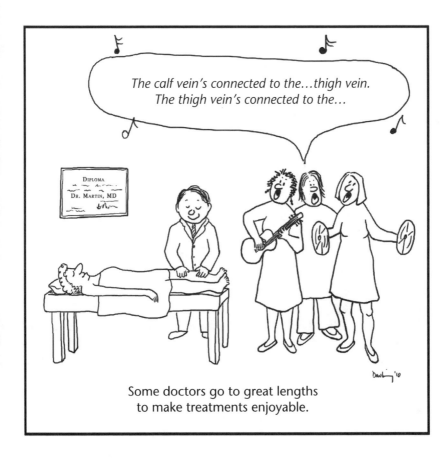

Some doctors go to great lengths
to make treatments enjoyable.

When treating vein disease, the big ones go first!
In other words, varicose veins and other larger veins with valve insufficiency problems should be treated before spider veins.
This sounds like common sense.
But in fact, improper sequencing of treatment is a common medical error in the real world.

After three sessions, our patients will usually experience about 90 percent clearing of spider veins and feeding green veins. An additional three treatments will typically increase the level of clearing to about 98 percent. Even if you have very severe spider veins, you should be able to achieve 95 to 99 percent clearing with a series of six treatment sessions.

After a series of six treatments, I like to stop for at least six months to give your body time to rest, and to allow the leg veins to adapt to the new blood-flow patterns. Your legs will continue to heal and clear for the next three to six months. For two to four months after the last treatment session is completed, their visual appearance will gradually improve.

Big ones go first

When treating vein disease, the big ones go first! In other words, varicose veins and other larger veins with valve insufficiency problems should be treated before spider veins. This sounds like common sense. But in fact, improper sequencing of treatment is a common medical error in the real world.

If spider vein problems are treated without first addressing the more major varicose vein problems, the spider veins will simply recur. In fact, treating spider veins without first resolving the bigger vein problems is like pouring gasoline on a fire. It can actually worsen the situation.

You'd be surprised how many patients have come to my office after having had multiple spider vein treatments with poor results and high rates of recurrence. In most cases their doctors made the mistake of treating their spider veins without first treating the larger incompetent veins. This is another reason why you should find an experienced vein specialist who will perform an assessment utilizing color-flow duplex ultrasound before initiating treatment.

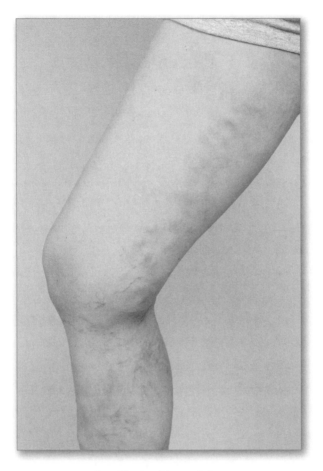

A patient with a mixture
of varicose and spider veins

Mopping up

After initial vein treatments with sclerotherapy, I typically use laser and in-tense pulse light (IPL) therapies to clear out the remaining spider veins.

Lasers are effective for touching up small spider veins that are difficult to treat with even the smallest needles. A laser delivers an intense, amplified beam of light directly onto the vein, burning it and causing it to seal. Over time, the ablated vein will wither and be absorbed by the body.

Betty Lewis's Story

Betty Lewis, age 60, is a debt collector with a credit union.

In high school I actually had pretty nice legs. But when I became an adult, I worked in retail stores where I would stand on concrete floors in high heels most of the day. That was hard on my legs. Getting pregnant and gaining weight didn't help. Over time, my legs began to look ugly. They felt hot and the pain was like a toothache.

After a few years, I got a job where I could sit most of the day, but that wasn't good for the circulation in my legs either. They got where they looked real bruised. My friends would say, "What have you done to your legs?"

A friend of mine had saline injections for her varicose veins, but they didn't help her. So I didn't think there was much hope for me, until I found out about Dr. Martin and scheduled an appointment. By that time I couldn't even walk up steps, and my legs definitely weren't pretty.

After the first treatment with Dr. Martin, my legs felt considerably better. I've had several follow-up treatments since then, and they keep improving. There's no more heat in my legs and no pain! I can walk up steps without any problem. My legs are not quite as pretty as they were in high school, but I'm very satisfied.

Many different types and wavelengths of lasers are effective in treating spider veins in the legs and in the face, but I prefer the Dornier 940-nanometer diode laser. It successfully seals and destroys spider veins without harming the nearby skin tissue, thus minimizing the risk of scarring or discoloration. This laser's wavelength has the ideal absorption rate in both the hemoglobin of red blood cells and the water of the vein walls.

Lasers can produce some mild discomfort that feels somewhat like the snap of a hot rubber band against the skin. To minimize this discomfort, I use a cooling device that blows refrigerated air against the skin's surface, partially numbing it. When working on facial spider veins, I often will also apply some numbing medication cream twenty to thirty minutes before treatment. Numbing creams are not normally used on the legs, however, because the legs are not as sensitive as the face. Also, very large dosages would be required.

Intense pulse light therapy (IPL), mentioned in the previous chapter, is another effective method for treating spider veins over a larger area. Like laser technology, it should only be used to treat spider veins if foam sclerotherapy is also used to treat the underlying feeding green veins.

The combination of laser and foam sclerotherapy can be very effective. Some doctors call it the "double injury approach," because it treats the veins with both light and chemicals.

Avoiding pigmentation problems

Laser and IPL treatments can cause patients with dark skin pigmentation or tans to have permanent, unsightly white or pink spots on the skin, as well as mild burns or blisters that can develop into scars. For this reason, I never use these therapies on African-American patients.

I use them on Hispanic or Asian patients only if they have been out of the sun for an extended period of time, or if they have unusually fair skin. In fact, I tell my Caucasian patients who are scheduled to undergo laser or IPL treatments to stay out of the sun and out of artificial tanning salons for at least a month prior to treatment.

Patients who have any type of skin disorder should discuss this with their physician during the initial evaluation. Some medications are light-sensitizing. Review your medication usage with your treating physician to reduce the risk of complications.

Saying Goodbye to Spider Veins

What to Expect after Sclerotherapy

YOUR SPIDER VEINS HAVE BEEN ATTACHED TO YOU FOR QUITE A WHILE—literally!—so they're going to be reluctant to say goodbye following treatment. Some of the very small ones may disappear instantly, but the medium-sized veins will take about two to six weeks to clear. Two to four months may be required for your body to clear the larger spider veins and the feeding green veins.

The best is yet to come

After sclerotherapy, your legs will look worse before they look better, especially if you're fair-skinned. But don't panic! The majority of the bruising and inflammation will subside within two weeks.

When planning your vein treatments, allow a reasonable amount of time for healing. Don't schedule a procedure two weeks before your beach vacation, for example. With sclerotherapy, "patients need patience."

For about a week after treatment, avoid submerging yourself in hot water. Warm showers are okay, but hot tubs and warm baths will cause your leg veins to dilate. For two to four weeks, avoid exposure to the sun.

We have our patients wear thigh-high or waist-high compression hose for one week after treatment. The compression is soothing, it accelerates clearing, and it minimizes bruising and inflammation. Compression hose also reduce the risk of complications due to trapped blood or phlebitis. For the first twenty-four hours, wear them continuously. During the next six days, you can remove them when retiring at night.

You will probably experience either no discomfort or very mild discomfort after spider vein treatment. Very mild burning or itching is temporary and okay. If some pain medication is desired, I usually recommend off-the-shelf remedies, such as Advil, Aleve, or Tylenol.

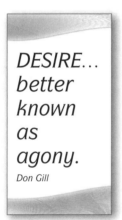

DESIRE...
better
known
as
agony.
Don Gill

To further accelerate the healing of bruises and mild tenderness associated with treatment, consider taking Arnica montana. It's a homeopathic medicine that is available from many stores that sell herbal remedies. As a convenience to patients, many vein specialists also offer it for sale in their offices.

It comes in an ointment version, but I prefer the tablets that dissolve under the tongue; they allow greater amounts of medication to enter the bloodstream. To minimize bruising and accelerate clearing of bruising and tenderness, we advise patients to start Arnica two days before treatment and continue using it for seven to ten days after treatment.

Heaven can wait

I want to warn you about an interesting phenomenon that I've noticed over the years. After spider vein treatments, a few patients—even some who are merely midway through a series of successful treatments and have already achieved 85 to 90 percent clearing of their abnormal leg veins—are disappointed with the results. Maybe that's because most of us have a tendency to minimize past imperfections and exaggerate present ones.

There seems to be a phenomenon that patients forget the size and prominence of the veins that previously disappeared with treatment. Once the old veins are "out of sight, out of mind," they become focused, almost obsessed, with the remaining visible veins on their legs. This is one reason why I typically recommend multiple treatment sessions.

I want to caution you in advance not to expect perfection. Although your vein treatments should produce significant improvement, you will never experience 100 percent clearing. God saved perfection for heaven.

I routinely take photographs of my patients' legs before and after treatment. If they express dissatisfaction, I show them the photographs. Often they are stunned when they see the "before" photos. It's amazing how many say something like, "I completely forgot how bad my legs used to look!"

My patients typically experience approximately 70 percent clearing of visual spider veins per session with an aggressive protocol. If you've had substantial spider veins on your legs, new ones will appear regardless of the quality or quantity of treatment sessions. However, proper treatment of feeding green veins will substantially reduce the rate at which new spider veins develop, as well as the quantity. So, you'll probably want to schedule occasional touch-up treatments at least every one to five years.

In the previous era, when we treated spider veins with hypertonic saline injections or laser alone, subsequent sessions were major procedures. We actually had to start over and re-treat the spider veins. In fact, it was not uncommon for the spider veins to be even worse than before. But times have changed! With modern spider vein protocols, touch-up sessions really are touch-up.

Ensuring that you're insured

Most commercial insurance carriers don't pay for sclerotherapy treatments for spider veins; they consider them to be cosmetic electives rather than medical necessities. I disagree with that decision for select patients, because spider veins can and often do cause pain, swelling, and other debilitating medical symptoms.

Fortunately, Medicare often covers sclerotherapy for spider veins when clinical symptoms are present and when more conservative treatment measures have proven unsatisfactory. Both Medicare and commercial insurance

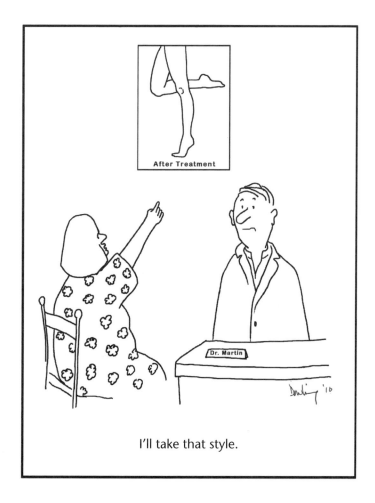

After Treatment

Dr. Martin

I'll take that style.

companies are more likely to give favorable consideration to spider vein cases when they also involve varicose veins or ultrasound abnormalities.

Insurance coverage can vary widely depending on the terms of the policies and the circumstances of each case. I advise discussing insurance issues with your vein specialist before starting treatment.

Sclerotherapy is one of the better values in surgery and medicine, even if you must pay for the procedure out of your own pocket. For a few hundred dollars, it can dramatically increase your body's energy and endurance, while reducing pain, swelling, restlessness, and other symptoms in your legs.

Sclerotherapy treatment of spider veins also can make you much better looking! For a relatively small investment, you can literally transform the basic appearance of your legs. People spend a lot more money on other types of cosmetic treatments for less dramatic results.

Improbable possibilities

Sclerotherapy is relatively safe. Side effects are usually minor and occur in only a small percentage of patients. But in the interest of full disclosure, and to give you a more comprehensive picture, I will mention a few.

Hyperpigmentation (staining)

In about 5 percent to 20 percent of patients, brownish splotches of discoloration can occur at the treatment site. If this happens to you, don't be alarmed. The stains will completely resolve and disappear, usually within three to twelve months.

What causes staining? One of the nurses on my staff has a good explanation that my patients can understand. She says it's caused by "old blood trapped in dead veins."

When the veins are sealed, some blood may remain in them. As the red blood cells in this trapped coagulum begin to break down, the hemoglobin produces a byproduct called hemosiderin. When this is absorbed into the deep layer of skin, it creates a brownish discoloration in fair-skinned patients, and a dark brown or blackish discoloration in individuals with darker skin.

Patients who have darker skin pigmentation, or very large and dense patches of spider veins, are somewhat more likely to experience staining. To minimize the risk for these patients, I will usually lower the concentration of the sclerotherapy injection agent.

If you experience staining and the discoloration does not disappear as rapidly as you would like, the trapped coagulum can often be drained though a simple needle puncture performed during the weeks after treatment. This maneuver, which is not as uncomfortable as it may sound, can prevent or minimize staining.

Months later, if needed, your physician can employ intense pulsed light (IPL) therapy, a technology that is frequently used to rejuvenate skin and eliminate sunspots, to accelerate the clearing process. In our practice, we offer these treatments to our patients at no additional charge.

Post-treatment superficial phlebitis

As injured veins are being absorbed into the body, the overlying skin occasionally will become inflamed, causing redness and warmth. Although this can look like an infection, it is actually a benign, self-limiting condition that rarely spreads up the leg or into the deep vein system. It has no relationship to the more dangerous deep vein thrombosis (DVT) or to other blood clot complications.

When patients have this condition, I usually advise wearing compression hose a few days longer than normal after treatment. It also helps to take ibuprofen or Advil for one to two weeks, until most of the inflammation and tenderness have subsided. Aspirin, which is a mild pain medication with anti-inflammatory and blood-thinning properties, also is effective.

Heat—applied by means of a warm washcloth or heating pad—can also sooth phlebitis, as can simply sitting in a tub of hot water. As with staining, a needle puncture to drain the trapped blood can relieve tenderness and promote healing.

Matting

As a result of sclerotherapy treatments, new patches of tiny red veins can sometimes develop on the surface of the skin. It's not clear what causes this "matting." It could be due to incomplete treatment of underlying feeding green veins or other deep veins with venous insufficiency problems. Or perhaps it's the body's way of relieving pressure as the flow of blood is being rerouted following sclerotherapy.

Whatever the cause, matting can be disturbing. After all, your goal was to get rid of spider veins, not swap them for new unsightly veins. To further complicate matters, matting often occurs after the first one or two sclerotherapy sessions, so you might initially assume, incorrectly, that additional treatments will worsen the situation. On the contrary, additional treatments generally improve the matting, while simultaneously clearing remaining spider veins.

The good news is that matting is a temporary condition. It usually clears up spontaneously within a few weeks, and it rarely lasts more than a year. Various medical techniques are also available to speed up the clearing process. Additional sclerotherapy, ohmic thermolysis, laser treatment, or intense pulse light (IPL) treatment can be helpful.

Ulcers

Sometimes ulcers a few millimeters in diameter (skin necrosis) can develop on the surface of the skin approximately two to five weeks after sclerotherapy treatment. It's not clear what causes them. Perhaps they occur when medication is injected into the vein with excessive pressure, so that it enters a neighboring connecting artery branch (arteriovenous fistula). Damage to a small artery could cut off the blood supply to a small patch of skin. Another popular theory is that sclerotherapy medicine leakage from veins or from needles damages the surrounding local tissue.

A topical antibiotic, such as Neosporin, applied two to three times daily will usually bring about healing within three to eight weeks. These ulcers, however, are more tender and painful and heal more slowly than their appearance and small size would indicate. They also can leave scars, but in most cases the scars are so small they're not disturbing. Nevertheless, if desired, larger scars can be removed under local anesthesia to improve appearance. Ulcers should be a rare complication in a quality vein practice.

Allergic reactions

Hives and other allergic reactions are uncommon. Severe allergic reactions to Sotradecol or polidocanol are rare. Patients with asthma are at greater risk for allergic reactions, and alternate methods might be considered if treatment is necessary.

Other rare but more serious side effects

- *Deep vein thrombosis (DVT)* caused by sclerotherapy is extremely rare. Walking and wearing compression hose immediately after treatment reduces this risk.

- *Strokes and mini-strokes* (formally known as *transient ischemic attacks*, or TIAs) are exceedingly rare. Only a few cases have been reported worldwide out of millions of treatment sessions. I mention them primarily to remind physicians to take extra precautions with patients who have cardiac disorders, such as septal defect (the layman's term is "hole in the heart"). Patients with a right-to-left heart shunt should not be treated with foam medication. Physicians can limit the risk of TIAs by diligently interviewing patients about their health status, carefully monitoring the volume of foam, and using carbon dioxide gas for making foam.

• *Intra-arterial injections* occur when the medical agent is inadvertently injected into an artery instead of into the vein. I have seen reports of cases with substantial complications, but they are rare.

Many of these potential side effects and complications are exceedingly uncommon. However, they can happen. So, minimize the risk by choosing a physician who is experienced in the treatment of vein diseases as a specialty, rather than someone who practices vein medicine as a sideline.

Aldine Crews' Story

Aldine Crews, age 65, is a retired pharmacy manager.

I've had leg-vein problems pretty much my whole life. Even as a teenager, my varicose veins bulged out and were very painful. Pregnancy made them much worse.

After each of my three children, I had vein-stripping operations. Every one of them was a terrible ordeal! I had to stay in the hospital for five days after the procedures, and then I had to keep off of my legs afterwards for six weeks or more. In addition, the surgeries were very painful.

You can understand why it took me so long to go back to another vein specialist. From time to time, I would have to see a doctor when I would get superficial blood clots in my left leg, but I kept putting off vein treatments.

Then I heard about Dr. Martin and decided to have him treat me. He and his staff have been wonderful. It's been great...a breeze! If I had known it was going to be this easy, I wouldn't have postponed treatments.

I've had three treatments on each leg, and the recovery has been smooth and quick every time. My legs feel much, much better! Recently I was on my feet from 9:00 a.m. to 6:00 p.m., and my legs didn't hurt at all.

What a blessing this has been! One of my daughters teased me recently and said she was going to buy me a miniskirt. I've never worn a miniskirt in my life, and I'm not going to start now. But I wouldn't be surprised if she bought me a bathing suit. If she does, I'm going to wear it!

Section Three

Varicose Veins: Diagnoses, Causes, and Treatments

CHAPTER TWELVE

The Comings and Goings of Varicose Veins

*How You Got Those Varicose Veins
and What You Can Do about Them*

HAVE YOU NOTICED ANY LARGE, BULGING VEINS ON YOUR LEGS? THOSE are varicose veins. Like spider veins, they are caused by chronic venous insufficiency (CVI). In other words, the culprits are leaky vein valves.

Varicose veins are typically more of a concern than spider veins, both medically and cosmetically. But, again, I have good news! The methods for treating varicose veins have dramatically improved in the last decade.

An experienced vein specialist usually should be able to clear those unsightly critters in a single treatment session. This is in contrast to spider vein therapy, which usually requires multiple treatments because we typically clear only about 70 percent of the abnormal veins in a single session.

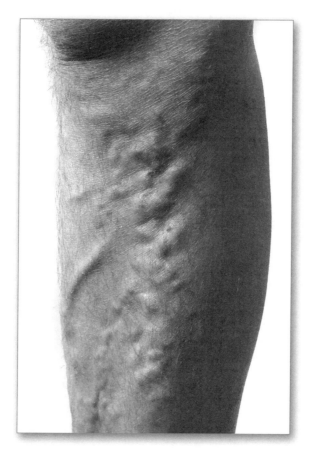

Varicose Veins

Good riddance

The vein-stripping and high-ligation surgery techniques that physicians used for many decades to treat varicose veins are now considered obsolete. Endovenous thermal ablation, typically performed in the physician's office under local anesthesia, has emerged as the new standard of care.

Endovenous thermal ablation destroys the veins that create chronic venous insufficiency, thus eliminating the problem at its source. Working with ultrasound guidance, the physician inserts a tiny heating element or laser filament into the insufficient leg vein through a very small catheter.

When the instrument is positioned in the target area, heat is applied to the interior aspect of the insufficient vein, damaging and sealing (ablating) it. The treated, or injured, vein turns into scar tissue. In succeeding weeks it is absorbed by the body.

After surgery, your body will automatically reroute the flow of blood through healthy veins. Over time, it will absorb the scar tissue from injured veins. You will enjoy improved circulation and better overall health.

Once gone, those varicose veins stay gone; modern treatment methods are remarkably durable. Prior to varicose vein procedures I often tell my patients, "Say goodbye to your abnormal veins. You won't see them again."

I will describe this endovenous thermal ablation procedure in more detail in subsequent chapters. But first, let's talk about how those varicose veins got there in the first place.

Britney Spears today is the equivalent of the average American woman—a single mother of two with dashed hopes, little faith in romance, and varicose veins.

The Varsity
October 12, 2007

Getting to the root of the problem

About 70 percent of major varicose vein problems originate in the great saphenous vein (GSV). That's the vein that runs from your groin area down your leg along your inner thigh to your knee and calf. From there it crosses your ankle onto the upper side of your foot.

The GSV is the longest vein in your body and the largest of the superficial leg veins. Its job is to collect blood from neighboring veins, which branch off of it much like the branches of a tree, and drain that blood up your leg back toward your heart.

Your GSV normally handles 3 to 5 percent of all the blood flowing in your leg. But it's a superficial vein, as opposed to a deep vein, because it resides in the fat layers of your leg, just above the muscular layers.

Despite its size, you don't need the GSV for proper circulation. That's why it's the vein most commonly harvested (removed) for coronary artery bypass surgery and for other vascular bypass procedures. Not only *can* you get by without your GSV, you are *better off* without it if it is not working properly.

In contrast, there's nothing superficial about your deep veins, which are deep in your muscles, toward the very center of your legs. They're the largest, most important veins in your legs, responsible for carrying about 90 percent of the blood up your legs and back to your heart. In all treatments for spider veins and varicose veins, we leave the deep vein system alone.

How varicose veins develop

To better understand how varicose veins develop, refer to illustration 12.1. Notice how your GSV branches off of the deep vein of your leg (the femoral vein) around groin level. That connection is called the saphenofemoral junction.

There's a one-way valve in your GSV just below the saphenofemoral junction. When the valve is working properly, it allows blood to flow efficiently upward through your GSV and into your femoral vein on its way to your heart, but not in the reverse direction.

However, if that valve is insufficient (leaky), some of the blood flowing upwards through your femoral vein will reflux into your GSV at the saphenofemoral junction. This will overwhelm the blood flowing upward through GSV and, aided by the force of gravity, will begin to push it back down the GSV. That's the wrong direction!

As if this weren't bad enough, the thin walls of your GSV will begin to expand (dilate) under the pressure of the refluxing blood, permitting more and more blood to enter your GSV from your femoral vein. There are about a dozen other valves in the GSV. The higher pressure, coupled with vein dilation, will cause progressively greater valve leakage further down the leg.

The weight of the blood due to the force of gravity causes vein pressures in the lower parts of the legs to increase. Your GSV is supposed to transport 3 to 5 percent of the blood in your legs *upward* toward your heart, as we have said. But a GSV that is dilated due to a leaky valve at the saphenofemoral junction typically carries 10 to 30 percent of the blood in your legs *downward*!

Your poor calf pump will now have to work a lot harder to move your blood up your legs. In fact, because a significant portion of your blood essentially is traveling in a circle, your body will have to pump some of the same blood over and over again.

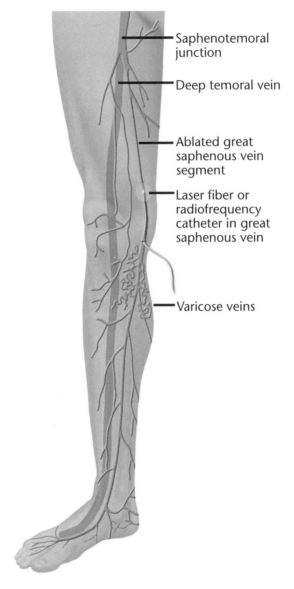

Saphenotemoral junction

Deep temoral vein

Ablated great saphenous vein segment

Laser fiber or radiofrequency catheter in great saphenous vein

Varicose veins

Fig 12.1 Typical placement of the catheter and treating device in the great saphenous vein.

The force of gravity

The refluxing blood accumulates under increasing pressure due to its own weight in the lower segments of your GSV and in the veins branching from it. Over the course of months and years, this pressure will stretch and eventually weaken the walls of these veins. That's how varicose veins develop in the lower parts of your legs, particularly around your inner knee, calf, ankles, and feet.

The GSV itself can dilate enough to become a visibly bulging varicose vein. However, most visible varicose veins are actually tributary veins branching off of your GSV. This process can cause inflammation and scarring in the legs and sometimes results in spider veins. A sedentary lifestyle with prolonged periods of sitting, or an occupation that requires much standing, will accelerate this debilitation.

Although the GSV is the source of 70 percent of the cases of varicose vein cases, other veins can cause problems, too. The remaining 30 percent of major varicose vein cases are due to insufficiencies in the tributary branches of the great saphenous vein; valve problems in the small (or lesser) saphenous vein, which branches from the deep veins behind the knee and proceeds down the back of the calf; and defects in a few other superficial veins. In fact, patients with varicose veins often have several defective veins and combinations of the above abnormalities.

Now you can understand why it's important to ablate, or destroy, an insufficient great saphenous vein. It's the head of the crime syndicate, the malevolent boss of the gang of troublemaking veins. Putting this culprit out of action is the most important step in eliminating varicose veins, because it attacks the root cause of the problem.

When venous reflux and chronic venous insufficiency problems are resolved, the remaining healthy veins are able to briskly move blood up your legs. In fact, getting rid of abnormal superficial veins (spider veins and varicose veins) actually takes stress off of the deep vein system by eliminating the recirculation of blood through the veins.

The endovenous ablation techniques discussed in the following chapters can be used to treat all of these veins. But for the sake of simplicity, I'll only describe the procedure we use for the GSV, since it's the most common source of problems.

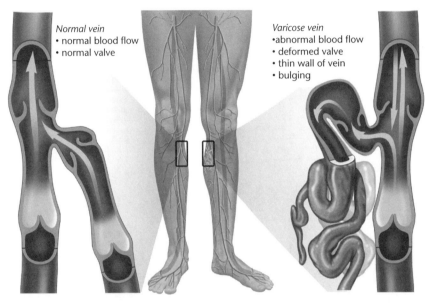

Normal vein
• normal blood flow
• normal valve

Varicose vein
•abnormal blood flow
• deformed valve
• thin wall of vein
• bulging

Fig. 12.2 How normal veins function (left) and how varicose veins develop from incompetent valves branching from an abnormal saphenous vein (right).

Shedding Light on the Problem

*State-of-the-Art Advances
in the Treatment of Varicose Veins*

IT'S A GOOD THING THAT THE VEIN-STRIPPING SURGICAL TECHNIQUES THAT once were the standard of care for varicose veins are now considered obsolete. One drawback was that they usually required a stay in a hospital or outpatient surgery center, which added considerably to the expense.

Secondly, these procedures required the use of general or spinal anesthesia. This further increased the costs, posed some additional risks, and lowered patients' post-operative energy levels. Because of the severity of the procedures, many patients could not return to work for several weeks.

Thirdly, these now-obsolete methods not infrequently involved considerable pain and left disfiguring leg scars. And finally, there was a surprisingly high rate of recurrence of disease. After all of this discomfort and inconvenience, patients stood as much as an 80 to 90 percent chance of getting varicose veins again sometime during their lifetime.

Fortunately, the situation has dramatically improved. The newer endovenous thermal ablation techniques, which typically utilize either laser or radiofrequency (RF) energy, offer a host of advantages over the old sclerotherapy and vein-stripping approaches. No doubt that's one reason why the treatment of leg-vein disease has become a booming field in the last decade.

Advantages of the new techniques

One major advantage of the new endovenous thermal ablation techniques is that they're usually performed in the physician's office under local anesthesia. This dramatically decreases costs, improves convenience, and shortens recovery time. It also reduces the risks associated with general anesthesia. Consequently, your physician can be much more comfortable treating you, even if you have minor heart problems or other health issues.

The newer techniques, which utilize needle puncture approaches working through very small catheters under ultrasound guidance, also involve considerably less discomfort during and after the procedure than the old vein-stripping procedures. And because they are minimally invasive, the risks of complications from wound infections, blood clots, and nerve injuries are significantly lower. Patients usually enjoy faster healing and a substantially improved cosmetic appearance, with virtually no scars.

By eliminating the need for a hospital stay and general anesthesia, the new endovenous thermal ablation techniques typically reduce overall costs to patients and insurers by more than 80 percent. With the previous methods, hospital and anesthesia fees comprised the largest portion of the costs of vein surgery, even for outpatients.

Last, but not least, the new endovenous thermal ablation techniques are much more durable. Studies show that they are successful five years after treatment for upwards of 90 percent of patients. In experienced, well-trained hands, the great majority of patients have an excellent likelihood of lifetime resolution of varicose veins and major venous insufficiency. That's in sharp contrast to the treatment methods of the previous era, where the recurrence of varicose veins was likely.

Ultrasound guidance has been a significant reason for this improved success rate. Before ultrasound was available, surgeons operated somewhat blindly. Occasionally they stripped the wrong vein. When patients had multiple veins with defective valves, physicians sometimes stripped one vein correctly but missed other defective veins.

I have heard estimates that, before the use of ultrasound, only 50 percent of vein-stripping operations were performed correctly and completely. This is not to criticize the surgeons of prior decades, but to point out the challenges they faced due to a lack of diagnostic information.

Today, diagnostic ultrasound helps physicians visually identify all defective leg veins with precision. Utilizing color-flow duplex ultrasound, we can even see the velocity and direction of blood flow through the veins. Ultrasound also serves as a quality-control instrument because it helps to assure that no abnormal veins will be missed; they have to be visualized by ultrasound as they are treated with the newer techniques.

The two major treatment technologies

Two modalities account for almost all varicose vein treatments performed in the United States where there is saphenous vein insufficiency: endovenous radiofrequency ablation (RFA) and endovenous laser treatment (EVLT).

RFA and EVLT are simply different ways of delivering heat to the internal aspect of the diseased saphenous vein. As we described in the preceding two chapters, the heating instrument is inserted through a catheter into the vein with the help of ultrasound guidance while the patient is under local anesthesia. The heat damages (ablates) the targeted section of the defective vein, causing it to close and seal.

These two methodologies are discussed in the remainder of this chapter. Although EVLT is the more popular method, I and most other treatment experts consider both techniques to be outstanding advances in the treatment of varicose veins and CVI.

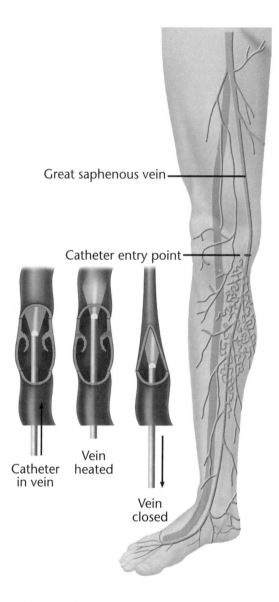

Great saphenous vein

Catheter entry point

Catheter
in vein

Vein
heated

Vein
closed

Fig. 13.1 The heating device is inserted through a catheter into the incompetent saphenous vein, and the applied heat closes the vein.

Endovenous radiofrequency ablation

Endovenous radiofrequency ablation (RFA) technology was first approved by the FDA in 1999. The original procedure, called VNUS Closure®, was developed by VNUS, Covidien. A radical improvement over previous methods of treating varicose vein disease, it has enjoyed a high technical success rate.

Endovenous RFA utilizes oscillating electrical energy generated by bipolar electrodes to transmit heat to the diseased vein. Placing the heating element in direct contact with the internal aspect of the wall of the insufficient vein causes it to collapse and seal. A feedback safety mechanism prevents temperatures from rising above 90°C.

The term *radiofrequency* indicates that the electrical energy produced by the instrument lies within the radio wavelength range. Initially RFA was a somewhat cumbersome and time-consuming procedure because the physician often had to make multiple passes with the instrument.

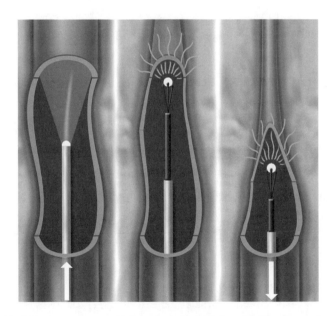

Fig. 13.2 Endovenous radiofrequency ablation (RFA) of a saphenous vein. The RFA heating device is inserted into the incompetent vein through a catheter *(left)*, heat is applied *(center)*, and the vein closes as the device is withdrawn *(right)*.

VNUS has since introduced the ClosureFAST RF ablation technique. It has considerably shortened treatment times while improving patient comfort. VNUS has also introduced the Closure RFS and Closure RFS flex thermal ablation devices for the treatment of perforator veins.

RFA techniques are developing a good track record for technical success, symptom relief, and improved quality of life for patients.

Endovenous laser ablation techniques

Since the first laser device was approved by the FDA in 2002, endovenous laser treatment (EVLT) has surged ahead of RFA in popularity. Today it accounts for almost 70 percent of all endovenous thermal ablations in the United States and about 85 percent worldwide, and these percentages continue to increase.

As mentioned in chapter 9, LASER is an acronym for Light Amplification by Stimulated Emission of Radiation. A laser amplifies a narrow (single-wavelength) beam of electromagnetic radiation (light energy) to create intense focused energy. Using a fiber-tipped EVLT device, the physician delivers energy directly to the wall of the diseased vein.

Physicians and other experts disagree about how to best use a laser for venous ablation. Some believe that the tip of the instrument should be placed in direct contact with the walls of the vein. Others think that the laser destroys the vein by heating the blood inside the wall, so that direct contact is not necessary. Regardless, both ablation methods are highly successful.

Early EVLT instruments utilized a bare-tipped fiber. More recently, some laser manufacturers have introduced covered-tip fibers, which substantially reduce discomfort, tenderness, and bruising. Advances have also been made with radial-tip fibers.

Since 2002, the FDA has approved laser instruments utilizing several different wavelengths: 810 nm, 940 nm, 980 nm, 1320 nm and, more recently, 1470 nm. A nanometer (abbreviated *nm*) is one billionth of a meter.

The new, longer-wavelength instruments, including the 1320 nm and 1470 nm, have a different physical pattern of energy of absorption. An advantage of the 1470 nm laser, for example, is that it has a greater absorption by water and a lesser absorption by hemoglobin. Only a fraction of the laser energy is required to successfully ablate the vein as compared to shorter wavelengths.

For many years, beginning in 2003, I used Dornier's 940-nm diode laser to perform thousands of successful ablation procedures. Some patients, however, experienced mild-to-moderate tenderness or bruising that required the use of Advil or Motrin for several days.

More recently, I've treated hundreds of patients with the Thermolite® 1470 nm diode laser, marketed by Total Vein Solutions. Most have experienced no more than very mild tenderness or bruising. Many of my patients do not even need Advil or Motrin.

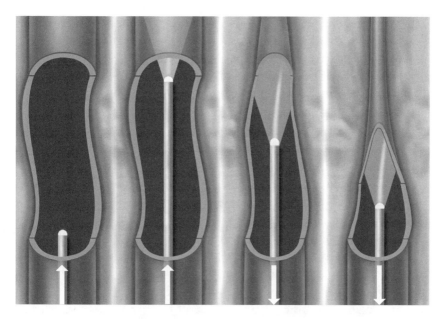

Fig. 13.3 Endovenous laser treatment (EVLT) of a saphenous vein. The laser heating device is inserted through a catheter into the incompetent saphenous vein and heat is applied. The vein closes as the device is withdrawn.

RFA vs. EVLT

Both radiofrequency and laser ablation techniques are safe and effective treatment methods in the hands of well-trained and experienced physicians. There have been anecdotal reports and informal discussions among physicians that radiofrequency ablation may somewhat increase the risk of nerve injuries, skin burns, deep vein thrombosis, or instrument defect. However, I'm unaware of any quality medical study that shows a statistical difference between RFA and laser technology with respect to safety or complications.

In the earlier years, RFA caused less tenderness and bruising than EVLT. However, the recent introduction of covered-tip and radial-tip laser fibers, along with longer-wavelength lasers, has narrowed this difference. I and several of my colleagues around the country consider 1470 nm diode laser ablation and RFA to be approximately equivalent in terms of post-operative comfort and recovery.

EVLT has in many studies tended to have a better long-term closure rate than RFA. A meta-analysis (a study of a compilation of many studies) has reported a saphenous vein closure rate for EVLT of 94 percent at the end of three years, while the closure rate for RFA was 84 percent.[11] To be fair, these studies involved the original VNUS Closure® technique. Future studies of the CloseFAST® technique of more recent years may show a narrowing of this gap.

Multiple companies manufacture laser instruments in the United States, while only one company manufactures radiofrequency instruments. Perhaps due in part to this competition, the costs of laser instruments and procedures are lower. Since the medical results from RFA and EVLT are similar, I suspect that the lower cost of EVLT is the major reason for its popularity with practitioners.

In my opinion, and in the opinion of some of my colleagues, lasers are more versatile and less cumbersome than RFA instruments. Because they can be more deftly manipulated, I often use them to treat smaller-caliber (narrower) veins and shorter segments of veins.

In conclusion, radiofrequency ablation (RFA) and laser ablation (EVLT) represent outstanding advances in the treatment of varicose veins and chronic venous insufficiency. Both techniques should be considered safe and effective when performed by a well-trained and experienced physician.

Possible new EVLT technology

In addition to the multiple wavelengths of lasers referred to above, I have heard discussion about research that is currently underway concerning the use of even higher wavelengths. I would not be surprised if in the future some of the wavelengths used for endovenous laser ablation approach or enter the infrared range of the electromagnetic spectrum.

The advantage of longer-wavelength lasers may be a further reduction in post-treatment tenderness and bruising, which could mean shorter, more comfortable recoveries for patients. They may also eliminate need for applying local anesthesia.

Clarivein

Clarivein is an emerging endovenous ablation method for treating varicose and saphenous veins. It holds significant promise as a more comfortable, less costly technique than some other procedures in current use. The Clarivein device has already been approved for use in Europe, and I suspect that it will be approved by the FDA for use in the United States.

This new technique is similar to the other procedures described above in that the treatment device (in this case a very small wire) is placed through a catheter into the insufficient vein utilizing ultrasound guidance and local anesthesia. A major advantage is that the numbing medication is not required around the vein because no thermal energy (heat) is applied.

As the device is withdrawn, the wire rotates briskly, roughing up (mildly injuring) the interior aspect of the vein wall. This makes the vein more susceptible to the sclerotherapy medicine that is infused through the catheter. The immediate vein closure (ablation) properties of this procedure are excellent. Studies will need to be performed to assess longer-term results.

---

11. R. van den Bos, L. Arends, et al. "Endovenous Therapies of Lower Extremity Varicosities: a Meta-Analysis," *Journal of Vascular Surgery*, 49 (2009): 230-9.

What's Up, Doc?

Varicose Vein Treatment Protocol

ARE YOU ONE OF THOSE ADVENTUROUS SOULS WHO THRIVES ON MYSTERY and uncertainty? Or do you prefer to know what you're getting into, especially when it involves your body?

If you're like me, it's the latter. So in the next two chapters, I'm going to put your mind at ease by telling you a bit about how varicose vein ablation procedures are performed. If you're contemplating varicose vein surgery, I think you will find this information helpful and reassuring.

In this chapter, I'll describe how endovenous thermal ablation procedures can go a long way toward eliminating varicose veins in your legs. In the next chapter, I'll tell you about some adjunctive procedures that I and other experienced vein practitioners use to supplement endovenous ablation to give our patients the most satisfying and complete results possible.

Going after the big, bad GSV

The FBI knows that the best way to put a crime syndicate out of commission is to go after the gang's boss. Likewise, the best strategy to rid of your legs of varicose veins is to go after the main

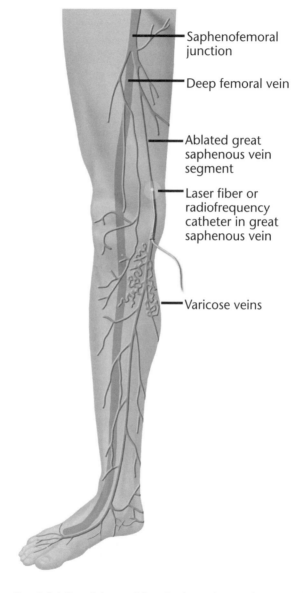

Saphenofemoral junction

Deep femoral vein

Ablated great saphenous vein segment

Laser fiber or radiofrequency catheter in great saphenous vein

Varicose veins

Fig. 14.1 Possible position for inserting catheter and heating device into incompetent saphenous vein.

culprit: your GSV (great saphenous vein). Although other veins are sometimes involved, getting rid of your GSV is usually far and away the most important step in getting rid of your varicose veins.

How do we do that? Well, we start by using ultrasound guidance to locate the veins to be treated. Once identified, we mark them on the skin's surface with a special felt-tip pen. I'll have you stand during this exam so gravity will pull the blood down into your defective veins, making them easier to see.

You may recall that we talked about ultrasound technology in chapter 7. Throughout the entire procedure, this invaluable tool helps us locate targeted veins and confirm the precise placement and positioning of instruments within the GSV.

Once the ultrasound exam is completed, we'll ask you to recline on the procedure table so a member of my medical team can paint the entire leg to be treated with a sterilizing solution and place sterile drapes and sheets around it. By the way, you're going to feel quite relaxed during this process because you will have taken a dose of prescription sedation medication ("chill pill" is our slang term for it) prior to coming to my office.

After numbing the skin with local anesthesia medicine, I use a needle and guide-wire system to insert a small-caliber catheter into your GSV. The entry level can vary, but it should be at the lowest point where blood reflux occurs, which is usually below the knee at the level of the upper calf.

Next, I'll pass the catheter upward through your GSV to the groin area of your leg. (This sounds like a bigger deal than it is! Most patients feel no discomfort.) Then I'll insert either a laser filament or a radiofrequency instrument through the catheter until it is positioned less than an inch below the groin junction of your GSV and your deep vein.

To ensure that you feel no pain when I ablate your GSV, I will now apply a significant volume of highly diluted numbing medication under gentle pressure around your GSV throughout the entire length to be treated. You will experience only minor discomfort—like slight pinches and pressure—when I introduce this medication.

The "magical" medicine

The numbing fluid that I use in this procedure, tumescent anesthesia medicine, is so marvelous that I want to take a moment here to tell you about it. I and many other vein specialists consider it nothing short of magical.

In addition to its excellent numbing qualities, the thick layer of tumescent anesthesia medicine around the saphenous vein simultaneously provides the following three outstanding benefits:

1. It pushes away neighboring nerves, arteries, muscle, and other structures, thereby protecting them from collateral heat damage.

2. It serves as an insulating heat sink that absorbs heat transmitted from the vein treatment area, further protecting the surrounding structures.

3. It prevents internal bleeding by exerting a gentle pressure around the veins being treated.

It would be difficult to exaggerate the importance of this remarkable medication. Without it, we probably would be unable to treat varicose veins with ablation techniques safely and efficiently in an office setting.

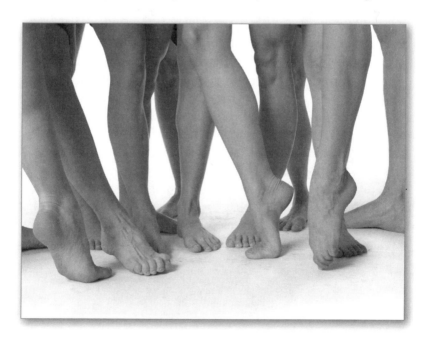

Putting the heat on

Now that we've located and numbed the chief culprit, it's time to turn up the heat by activating the laser (or the radiofrequency device). As the instrument is slowly withdrawn, the heat it generates will destroy (ablate) your GSV from its internal aspect. The flow of blood through your GSV will stop immediately, so that reflux (valve leakage) can no longer occur. Remember, this is virtually painless because of that miraculous tumescent anesthesia medicine.

Then another amazing thing happens! Your body immediately redirects blood from the destroyed GSV and its connecting tributary veins to neighboring normal veins that have properly functioning valves.

At this point we have taken a giant leap toward restoring God's original design for your body. The veins in your legs are once again efficiently returning blood to your heart. Your body won't miss your defective GSV one bit. If fact, it will be as delighted as you would be if a gorilla with an insatiable appetite had decided to leave your home!

At the completion of treatment, I'll withdraw the catheter and the treatment instruments through the needle site in your skin. During the weeks following treatment, your destroyed saphenous vein will convert to scar tissue and your body will absorb it.

Back to the future

After state-of-the-art endovenous thermal ablation treatment for varicose vein disease, you should be able to get back to your normal routine in no time. But there's one big difference. The life you go back to promises to have a much more comfortable, enjoyable, and healthy future!

In the initial hours after a procedure, I encourage patients to walk while wearing elastic compression hose. This promotes good flow of the vein blood and minimizes the risk of blood-clot problems.

You typically will be able to engage in light activities immediately after surgery and return to work in one to two days. You may even be able to engage in vigorous exercise in one to two weeks. However, I strongly recommend that you avoid exposure to the sun for two weeks following treatment.

Lori McRae's Story

Lori McRae, age 35, is a patient care technician in a dialysis center.

When I had my first child about two and a half years ago, spider veins and varicose veins appeared on my right leg, and my left leg developed spider veins. It was painful. My job requires me to stand on my feet pretty much all the time, and at the end of the day my legs ached.

They also swelled up and looked pretty awful. I was embarrassed to wear shorts or swimsuits. Even though I was young, I figured I would have to wear jeans and long pants for the rest of my life.

Health problems were kind of new to me. Before my pregnancy, I used to jog quite a bit and do aerobics at a local gym.

I didn't like being unhealthy and in pain, so when someone referred me to Dr. Martin, I went in for an evaluation and eventual treatment.

The procedure was simple and relatively painless. On my first visit, he took care of the varicose and spider veins in my right leg. On the second visit, he cleaned up the spider veins in my left leg. The recovery was quick. I was back at work and doing other normal activities within two days.

My legs look and feel a whole lot better. I have no pain at all now. My self-confidence has come back, and I'm very comfortable wearing shorts and swim suits.

Mopping up action

We've now taken care of the boss of the crime syndicate: the GSV. But what about all of his henchmen who are still at large—those nasty varicose veins that branch off from the saphenous vein?

Well, some of them will spontaneously shrink, now that we've eliminated the source of the refluxing blood. A few of the smaller varicose veins may even disappear. About 20 percent of patients will be satisfied with the results of this initial treatment, so this is where many physicians stop.

However, about 80 percent of my patients are not happy when so many varicose veins are still "at large." Neither am I. Those lingering varicose veins are aesthetically unpleasing, and they can cause pain, swelling, and even blood-clot problems. There's no need for you to continue to suffer this risk and discomfort.

That's why I and many other experienced vein specialists perform supplementary procedures to surgically remove varicose veins during or following the saphenous vein ablation procedure. I'll talk about these adjunctive procedures in the next chapter.

Finishing in Style

Supplementary Procedures for Treating Varicose Veins

IT'S TIME TO CELEBRATE! WITH THE AID OF YOUR PHYSICIAN, YOU HAVE won a major battle. Harnessing the power of endovenous thermal ablation, you've put the great saphenous vein and some of the ugly, unhealthy varicose veins that branch off of it out of commission. That was priority #1 in your fight to say goodbye to varicose veins.

But the battle may not quite be won. You may still have residual bulging varicose veins if endovenous thermal ablation of the saphenous vein was the only procedure performed. Can't something be done about them?

Going the extra mile

The answer is yes! Well-trained, experienced vein practitioners have some clever ways to get rid of these remaining bad guys. Three of the most common techniques are

- ambulatory microphlebectomy,
- foam sclerotherapy, and
- perforator vein ablation.

I'll tell you about these supplementary procedures and their benefits in a moment. But first, you may be wondering: If these supplementary procedures are so necessary and beneficial, why don't all vein practitioners perform them?

Frankly, some vein practitioners simply don't have the training and experience to offer these adjunctive procedures. This is especially true of physicians who try to learn how to ablate the saphenous vein in weekend workshops, with the goal of using vein surgery to supplement their practice income.

Over the years, I've treated hundreds of patients who were unhappy with the results of endovenous ablation procedures performed by less-experienced physicians. Most of these patients still suffered unnecessarily from pain, swelling, unsightliness, and other symptoms of vein disease. Their veins persisted and worsened; some recurred worse than before.

That's why I strongly encourage you to find a well-trained, experienced physician who practices vein surgery as a specialty, not merely as a sideline. Make sure your doctor has the capability to perform the adjunctive procedures described in this chapter. When evaluating vein practitioners, this capability separates the best from the rest. (In my less enlightened days, I might have said it separates the men from the boys!)

Can both be right?

There are two schools of thought about if and when to perform these adjunctive procedures. Some physicians believe it's best to wait for two to three months after the initial endovenous ablation treatment. Other equally competent physicians favor performing the adjunctive procedures concurrently with the endovenous treatment. Which school of thought is right?

Actually, they both are. Or perhaps it's more accurate to say that neither approach is wrong. I'll give you some of the arguments in favor of each. Then I'll divulge my personal bias.

The first school of thought—allowing two to three months to pass before performing adjunctive procedures—is considered by some to be the more conservative approach. "About 20 percent of patients will be satisfied with the initial treatment," say physicians who subscribe to this view. "It's overly aggressive to perform supplementary procedures on 100 percent of patients, when only 80 percent will want or need them."

"What's more, smaller varicose veins will resolve on their own during this waiting period, and the larger varicose veins will shrink, " these practitioners point out. "Letting a little time pass ensures that additional procedures, if and when they are performed, will be less extensive."

"You've overlooked some important considerations," counter physicians who subscribe to the second school of thought. "During this two- to three-month waiting period, patients may continue to needlessly suffer from pain, swelling, and other symptoms of vein disease. Abnormal clusters of varicose veins are left behind and will persist in 80 percent of cases, and patients are certain to be unhappy with the appearance of their legs. So, why wait?"

"Furthermore," physicians in this second school might continue, "while patients are waiting for further treatments, blood can collect in the remaining varicose veins, possibly causing blood clots. Although superficial thrombophlebitis is not life-threatening, it certainly can be a painful nuisance. And in about 15 percent of cases, it may propagate into the deep vein system, where it can become the more dangerous deep vein thrombosis."

My personal bias

Since there is no established protocol or standard of care at this time, I'll give you my personal bias: I'm firmly in the second camp. I favor performing these supplementary techniques concurrently with endovenous thermal ablation.

Since 80 percent of patients will need or desire additional treatments to resolve their varicose vein disease anyway, I see no reason to postpone treatments and thereby unnecessarily subject these patients to risks of blood clots. Performing adjunctive procedures concurrently with endovenous ablation requires very little additional time. And because the procedures are minimally invasive, the risk of complications is extremely small.

Concurrent procedures offer patients the following significant benefits:

- Increased satisfaction following the initial procedure
- Greater immediate resolution of varicose vein problems
- Reduced risk of blood-clot complications
- Reduced medical fees because all procedures are done in one session
- Less time away from work because there are fewer treatment sessions

Insurance considerations may dictate the timing of adjunctive procedures. Some policies require that conservative treatment measures (e.g., elevation of the legs, wearing compression hose, and taking pain medications) be tried before additional procedures will be approved. This can be frustrating for patients and physicians.

Now that we've discussed the timing issue, I'll tell you a bit about each of the three most common supplementary procedures.

Ambulatory microphlebectomy

Microphlebectomy is a popular technique in which varicose veins are removed through tiny nick incisions using a very small instrument that is somewhat like a miniature crochet hook. It's called "ambulatory" microphlebectomy because patients often can be lightly active immediately after the procedure.

The small incisions—about 1 to 2 mm in length—leave virtually no scars. They heal beautifully without stitches or butterfly tape. In fact, I and some of my colleagues are now able to remove most varicose veins through a needle puncture.

Microphlebectomy is performed under local tumescent anesthesia. Large volumes of diluted numbing solution are injected just under the skin around the varicose veins, so you'll experience no more than mild tenderness following this procedure. In experienced hands, the cosmetic results are outstanding and nearly scarless.

I wanted to insert a warning about a technique often referred to as powered phlebectomy, or Trivex phlebectomy. This procedure uses a device to suction out varicose veins through relatively small incisions in the skin. A "Roto-Rooter" type of rotating blade in the device morselizes the varicosities as they are removed.

This technique has fallen out of favor with the vascular surgery and phlebology communities because it generally has to be done in an operating room setting with anesthesia. Furthermore, it leaves scars that are generally small, but can be visible, and it involves a greater risk of nerve injuries and chronic pain problems after treatment.

I don't mean to criticize expert practitioners who use this technique, as it can be an improvement over the old vein-stripping procedures. However, if your doctor recommends this technique, make sure he or she has had considerable experience and good results with it.

Foam sclerotherapy

The microphlebectomy procedure discussed above works well on larger, bulging varicose veins. But for removing small to mid-size veins, I and many of my colleagues prefer foam sclerotherapy. It is even less invasive than microphlebectomy, and for smaller veins it poses an even lower risk of side effects.

The foam medication—usually Sotradecol or polidocanol—is injected directly into the abnormal veins, causing them to close and ultimately disappear. For guidance in needle placement, I typically use a transilluminating vein light that gives a bright orange glow to the skin and fat tissue. When the lights in the room are dimmed, the veins show up as very dark lines under the skin.

Perforator vein ablation techniques

You may recall from chapter 8 that perforator veins are the short, connecting bridge veins that carry blood from your superficial vein system to your deep vein system. Each perforator vein has one valve. If it becomes defective, blood can flow in the reverse (wrong!) direction, causing varicose and spider veins to develop. For complete healing of varicose veins, you need to get rid of incompetent perforator veins. If you don't, they also can cause local skin and tissue damage and even open wounds (venous stasis ulcers).

There's disagreement, however, about if and when to treat incompetent perforator veins. Some physicians prefer to allow some time to pass after treatment for varicose veins. If rashes, inflammation, or other complications develop (some common medical terms for these conditions are venous stasis ulcers and venous stasis dermatitis), these physicians will then treat the perforator veins that seem to be causing the problems. They will also consider perforator vein ablation if varicose veins recur.

On the other hand, I and some of my colleagues favor treating all abnormal leg veins, including defective perforator veins, during the initial or subsequent treatment session in order to resolve as much venous insufficiency as possible. The exact indications for the treatment of incompetent perforator veins has yet to be defined by medical experts and research.

Popular treatments for perforator veins

The two most popular techniques for treating perforator veins are ultrasound-guided foam sclerotherapy (UGFS) and endovenous thermal ablation. Two previous methods—the Linton procedure (open surgery that involves tying off and dividing incompetent perforator veins) and the SEPS procedure (subfascial endoscopic perforator surgery that is done through small incisions and requires general anesthesia and a hospital stay) are increasingly considered obsolete.

My favorite method is ultrasound-guided foam sclerotherapy (UGFS). Because perforator veins are too deep to be seen with the eye, I use ultrasound to guide the placement of the needle or catheter. A higher concentration of foam sclerotherapy medicine is then injected into the abnormal perforator veins so they seal and eventually wither away.

The other increasingly popular technique for treatment of perforator veins is endovenous thermal ablation using either a laser or a radiofrequency instrument. This is essentially a smaller-scale version of the technique as described in chapter 14 for treating the great saphenous vein.

You should be able to resume your normal activities immediately after either ultrasound-guided foam sclerotherapy (UGFS) or endovenous thermal ablation. Wearing compression hose for a time after treatment will promote healing.

Some physicians who practice vein surgery as a sideline do not have the capability to perform the above procedures. That's why it's important to find an experienced, well-trained vein specialist.

TIRS technique for healing venous ulcers

Dr. Ron Bush, director of the Midwest Vein & Laser Center in Dayton, Ohio, has recently introduced an interesting new treatment concept to accelerate the healing of venous stasis ulcers. These ulcers, mentioned earlier in this book, develop in the lower legs and ankles and are notoriously stubborn to heal.

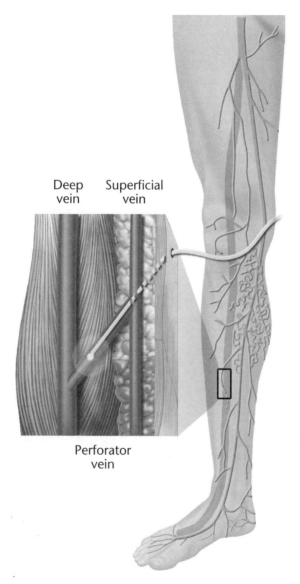

Deep vein   Superficial vein

Perforator vein

Fig. 15.1 Ablation of a perforator vein.

It is not uncommon for venous stasis ulcers to persist for many months – perhaps as long as one to three years – even when appropriate leg elevation, compression therapy, and wound-care methods are applied. They also have a rather strong tendency to recur after they have previously healed.

Dr. Bush has proposed a treatment concept he calls Terminal Interruption of the Reflux Source (TIRS).[12] Using ultrasound guidance, the vein specialist physician will identify any large incompetent vessels just beneath the wound area. Then, with the use of numbing medication and ultrasound guidance, a higher concentration of Sotradecol foam will be injected into a perforator vein or into an enlarged incompetent venous branch just beneath the wound.

TIRS reduces the pressure produced by the incompetent vein. In most cases, the wound will heal in just a few weeks. Definitive treatment for any other venous insufficiency problem, such as saphenous vein ablation, can be carried out in subsequent weeks and months for greater long-term resolution of venous insufficiency in the leg.

---

12. RG Bush, "New Technique to Heal Venous Ulcers: Terminal Interruption of the Reflux Source (TIRS)," *Perspectives in Vascular Surgery and Endovascular Therapy* 22(3): 194 – 199. 2010

Section Four

Conclusion

Looking Forward

What to Expect after Your Treatments

CONGRATULATIONS! IF YOU'VE UNDERGONE THE STATE-OF-THE-ART TREAT-
ments for vein disease described in this book, you're no doubt
looking forward to a healthier, more energetic life. But exactly what
long-term results can you expect? And what steps should you take
to maintain your improved level of health?

I'll answer these questions separately for spider veins and varicose veins, since there are significant differences between them.

Spider vein follow-up

After the initial three to six treatments for spider veins, your legs
should be 95 to 99 percent clear of visible disease. That's an amazing result! And to add to the good news, you should maintain a
high level of clearing for the rest of your life.

However, due to the normal aging process and the constant pull
of gravity, those nasty spider veins will constantly be trying to climb
back onto your legs. Also, you obviously are genetically predis-
posed to have vein disease, or you wouldn't have had problems in
the first place.

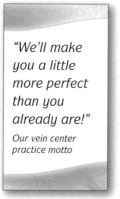

"We'll make you a little more perfect than you already are!"

Our vein center practice motto

So, you should not be surprised if some new spider vein problems develop. But because of the lasting effects of your initial treatments, you'll have about 85 percent fewer problems than you otherwise would have had. I'm sure you'd rather not have any new spider veins at all. But since perfection isn't possible, 15 percent sure beats 100 percent!

To ensure that your legs will look and feel great throughout your life, schedule occasional touch-up sessions with your vein specialist. If you originally had severe vein problems, I recommend an annual checkup. If you had a rather mild case of spider veins and you experienced excellent clearing with the initial sessions, touch-ups every three to five years should be fine.

Actually, "touch-up" is probably an inadequate term. Because these follow-up treatments utilize the same techniques as your initial treatments, the results will be just as comprehensive and durable. They don't simply shore up your prior treatments; they build on them.

During follow-up sessions, your physician should examine your legs and consider the need for ultrasound examinations. Any problematic spider veins or feeding green veins can be treated with sclerotherapy injections. Lasers or radiofrequency (ohmic) thermolysis might be appropriate for very small spider veins that are difficult to inject.

Varicose vein follow-up

If you suffered from varicose veins, your specialist probably used endovenous thermal ablation to treat your saphenous and perforator veins. In addition, you may have undergone microphlebectomy, foam sclerotherapy, or other procedures to rid your legs of varicose and spider veins.

As a result of improved circulation due to these treatments, you might have noticed that your legs feel lighter and fresher, and that you have greater physical endurance. Perhaps some or all of the heaviness, pain, swelling, cramps, and restlessness in your legs has disappeared. And certainly you must take comfort in knowing that your risks of phlebitis and blood clots have diminished.

All this is terrific! So, what can you expect going forward? What should you do to maintain your health?

Great expectations

Following the initial treatments, you can expect to have a 90 to 95 percent chance of being free of varicose veins for the rest of your life. That's a huge improvement over the results of treatments in prior eras! However, you still have a 5 to 10 percent chance of recurring disease. (A strong genetic tendency toward varicose veins pushes the risk toward the upper end of this range.) So let's talk about some preventive steps you can take.

Most new varicose veins will appear during the first two years after your initial treatment. Therefore, I suggest scheduling two to three checkups with your vein specialist during this two-year period. The more serious your chronic venous insufficiency and varicose vein disease problems were, the more frequently you should see your doctor.

Each visit should include an evaluation and examination utilizing surveillance ultrasound. Your physician will especially want to ensure that all of your previously treated veins have remained closed. Although ablated veins rarely reopen, it pays to be safe.

After endovenous ablation, your body reroutes the flow of blood in your legs. This process can occasionally put stress on other veins, and in 5 to 10 percent of patients it might cause leakage. If you do need subsequent treatment, your vein specialist can perform minimally invasive in-office procedures under local anesthesia with ultrasound guidance.

With state-of-the-art treatment methods, you probably won't need to schedule additional exams beyond two years, unless you have severe or complicated venous disease, or you desire follow-up spider vein therapy. If specific problems surface, simply call your doctor.

Saying goodbye

Most of us don't like goodbyes. Funerals, geographic relocations, job changes—even happy occasions such as graduations and weddings—can be emotionally stressful. But saying goodbye to varicose and spider veins is just the opposite. It's pure joy!

That's why I'm on a mission to tell you and everyone else about the revolutionary new methods for treating leg-vein disease. I want you to experience the happiness of saying goodbye to unhealthy, unsightly veins.

What a privilege it is to bring such good news. I like this mission!

What I Haven't Told You

Additional Information about
Vein Disease for the Exceptionally Interested

IT'S NOT UNCOMMON FOR MEDICAL STUDENTS TO BE FASCINATED BY UN-common, severe diseases. But my fellow students and I were taught that, when evaluating patients, less dramatic diagnoses are usually more accurate and common. One of our professors used to say, "If you hear hoofbeats on the ground outside your window, it could be a zebra, but it's more likely a horse."

This book is about horses; I've intentionally limited its scope to basic information about the causes and cures of varicose and spider veins. But for those of you who want to know about zebras, I've included the following information about some venous insufficiency conditions that are less common, but still important.

Acute deep venous thrombosis (DVT)

Acute DVT unfortunately is a fairly common medical condition, with up to 250,000 cases reported annually in the United States.

This is an emergency condition that involves the development of a blood clot in the deep veins of the leg. The most common symptoms are leg pain, swelling, redness, and warmth, typically occuring in one leg.

Some risk factors for DVT include smoking, use of oral contraceptives, hormone therapy, having a cancerous condition, undergoing major surgery and anesthesia, and prolonged periods of immobilization, such as after a major injury or illness. Also, the presence of a hypercoagulable state (see #4 below) can create an excessive tendency to form blood clots.

Acute deep vein thrombosis can also result in the more serious pulmonary embolism (see #2 below) or the development of post-thrombotic syndrome (see #3 below). Acute DVT is a true medical emergency. Patients who have unusual redness, pain, or swelling in one leg should see a physician or present to an emergency room as soon as possible. If acute DVT is the diagnosis (usually confirmed by an ultrasound exam), immediate use of blood-thinning medication usually will be prescribed, along with possible hospitalization.

Pulmonary embolism (PE)

PE is the most serious complication of deep vein thrombosis. It is known to occur in at least 10 percent of deep vein thrombosis cases, and there is reason to suspect that many more cases are not diagnosed because patients do not exhibit substantial symptoms.

PE constitutes a true dire medical emergency. Patients suspected of having this condition should immediately see a physician or, even better, present to an emergency room. Symptoms include shortness of breath and chest pain that becomes more severe with deep breathing.

PE occurs when a larger fragment of a blood clot breaks off from the deep veins of the leg, or from the pelvic veins, and travels in the bloodstream through the right side of the heart, ultimately blocking the arteries that transport blood to the lungs. A diagnosis of PE should be considered anytime a patient experiences sudden shock or a drop in blood pressure.

PE is the most common preventable cause of hospital deaths. Several professional medical societies are undertaking initiatives to improve prevention and treatment for deep vein thrombosis and, consequently, pulmonary embolism. Medical professionals and hospitals are taking steps to reduce the risk of PE for surgery patients, especially those having major surgery and general anesthesia.

Post-thrombotic syndrome (PTS)

PTS is a subsequent manifestation or complication of DVT. Often damage to the deep veins of the legs causes inflammation, scar tissue, and deformity to occur in the leg valves. This often results in a state of ongoing chronic venous insufficiency in the deep vein system, frequently in conjunction with the superficial venous system.

Symptoms include chronic leg pain, swelling, hyperpigmentation, scarring of the skin and fat around the lower leg, and possible ulcerations or wounds. Scarring related to previous blood clots in the veins can cause obstruction in the veins.

The usual conservative treatment measures (e.g., elevating the legs and using compression devices, such as graduated elastic compression hose) are especially important in treating PTS. Symptoms may be ameliorated by using some of the techniques described in this book for ablating incompetent saphenous veins and perforator veins and for treating varicose veins.

A vein specialist should be able to diagnose this condition and help arrange for appropriate evaluation and treatment. Patients with DVT high in the groin and pelvis levels should be considered for special treatment to dissolve and remove the clot (pharmacomechanical thrombolysis) and to help reduce the risk of subsequent PTS. These procedures are done via small catheters with x-ray guidance.

Hypercoagulable states

The term *hypercoagulable states* (or *thrombophilia*) covers a myriad of different diseases that typically involve some blood-clotting imbalance. Patients with these medical conditions often form blood clots more readily than normal, which increases their risk for deep vein thrombosis, pulmonary embolism, and superficial thrombophlebitis.

There is much medical science does not know about these complex diseases. However, some are known to be transmitted genetically. Smoking and taking oral contraceptives are causative and additive factors. Patients who have an unexplained blood clot, recurrent blood clot problems, or a family history of blood-clotting abnormalities should be tested for these diseases, even if they are young and healthy.

Stenosis or blockage of the iliac veins

The iliac veins, which are in the pelvic region, carry blood from the femoral leg veins to the inferior vena cava on its way back to the heart. Some patients, especially those who have had previous deep vein thrombosis, can incur a blockage or a severely narrowed vein (stenosis) in this area.

An experienced and alert vein specialist should be able to recognize this condition. It can become apparent either when an acute deep vein thrombosis develops that is related to poor blood flow, or when there is reflux of valves and chronic venous insufficiency in the legs.

May-Thurner syndrome is a variation of this condition that can especially occur in young women when the left iliac vein is compressed by an overlying iliac artery. This can result in obstruction and deep vein thrombosis. There can even be blockages in the inferior vena cava itself, which is the main vein draining blood from the lower half of the body.

Alert vein specialists are able to identify these conditions with magnetic resonance imaging (MRI) or other x-ray contrast studies performed through catheters (venograms). An interventional radiology specialist with x-ray guidance can place instruments across the obstruction, open it with a balloon dilation procedure (angioplasty), and place a stent (a small cylinder-shaped metallic cage device) to help maintain the vein in an open position.

Superficial thrombophlebitis (STP)

STP occurs when a blood clot forms in the superficial veins, which are all of the veins in the skin and fat layers, as well as those outside the muscle compartments. The superficial veins are the ones we most commonly treat for varicose and spider veins, as we have discussed in this book. Symptoms of STP can include sudden development of local tenderness and firmness over previous spider or varicose veins, along with local swelling and redness.

Patients with varicose veins or a hypercoagulable state have an elevated risk for developing STP. Contusions or other damage to the skin (e.g., from an IV catheter), aging, obesity, smoking, and the use of oral contraceptive medications can also increase the risks.

STP is considered more benign (less dangerous) than deep vein thrombosis (DVT). In approximately 14 percent of cases, however, it can propagate through connecting saphenous tributary or perforator veins into the deep vein system and cause DVT. For this reason, I recommend that patients with superficial thrombophlebitis have a thorough ultrasound examination of the leg to document the diagnosis, assess the extent of the thrombophlebitis, and make sure the clot has not traveled into or close to the deep veins.

Initially, treatment for STP might include the use of anti-inflammatory pain medications or aspirin, along with leg elevation measures and the use of graduated elastic compression hose. Once the condition has subsided, I advise patients to be evaluated for chronic venous insufficiency as well. If varicose veins or other variations of superficial venous insufficiency are present, they may be treated with endovenous ablation techniques or sclerotherapy, as described earlier in this book.

If the clot migrates to the groin area where the great saphenous vein connects with the deeper femoral vein, the patient is at very substantial risk of DVT and subsequent pulmonary embolism. Temporary use of blood-thinning medications is usually advisable. Ultrasound-guided surgical techniques should be considered to ligate the great saphenous vein to keep clots from spreading or migrating. Other treatments to address varicose vein issues may also be warranted. Again, I want to emphasize the importance of having an experienced and well-trained vein specialist treat these conditions.

Chronic deep vein insufficiency

In this book we primarily discussed *superficial* chronic venous insufficiency typically associated with varicose and spider veins. Although these are the most common manifestations of chronic vein insufficiency, a smaller percentage of patients can also develop chronic *deep* vein insufficiency, either alone or in combination with superficial venous insufficiency.

The typical symptoms of chronic deep vein insufficiency are very stubborn leg swelling and pain, possibly accompanied by skin ulcerations and soft-tissue scarring and discoloration. This condition is much more difficult to treat than superficial venous insufficiency because it involves the deeper veins of the legs, including the femoral, popliteal, and tibial veins. It can be present from birth (congenital), and it can also be caused when the valves are damaged or distorted due to inflammation or scarring from a previous blood clot disease, usually from acute deep vein thrombosis.

If patients suffer from both superficial and deep venous insufficiency, I join many other vein specialists in recommending aggressive treatment of the superficial venous insufficiency problem using the procedures described in this book. Frequently, but not invariably, these treatments will either resolve or improve the deep venous insufficiency problem by taking pressure off of the deep vein system.

If conservative treatment measures (e.g., leg elevation and compression therapy using leg hose or other devices) are not successful in treating the chronic deep vein insufficiency, consideration should be given to either transplanting or reconstructing the valves of the deep vein system or placing prosthetic valves. These procedures are typically done in highly specialized centers for patients with severe debilitating disease that are not relieved by other measures. I would refer such patients from my practice to a handful of surgeons around the United States who have experience with these types of operations.

Lymphedema

Lymphedema refers to a cluster of different conditions that involve swelling of the leg due to an abnormal flow of tissue fluid through lymph vessels.It can sometimes be severe, deforming, and disabling. Lymphedema is not a venous disease, but I include it here because it is a condition that causes swelling of the legs.

Lymph vessels, which are very small vessels located throughout the body, are quite dense in the legs. Their role is to collect body tissue fluid and proteins and to bring them back up through the legs toward the chest, where they drain into a large vein. Along the way, the lymph vessels pass through lymph nodes located in various parts of the body, such as behind the knee and very prominently in the groin region.

These lymph nodes harbor several types of very active white blood cells. Because they filter the lymph fluid to remove bacteria and foreign bodies, they are prone to collect cancer cells.

Lymphedema is not precisely understood. It could be the result of a flow phenomenon, abnormalities in very small valves within the lymph vessels, or other types of obstructions in the lymph vessels. Some physicians think that leg swelling in obese patients is due to mild lymphedema.

Patients with lymphedema are at higher risk for recurring infections, skin abnormalities, and wound problems. Because lymphedema is very difficult to cure, physicians typically focus on controlling the symptoms through very aggressive leg elevation and compression measures. Massage or compression pump devices used daily can sometimes help.

When patients have both venous insufficiency and lymphedema, treating the venous insufficiency with the techniques described in this book may help to control the lymphedema. But it should be emphasized that treatments for venous conditions in patients with lymphedema entail increased risks for patients. Again, it's important to consult an experienced vein specialist or vascular surgeon for treatment of this disease.

Klippel-Trenaunay Syndrome (KTS)

KTS is a rare congenital disorder that occurs when the patient is born with malformed blood vessels, typically in one leg. It often manifests itself as a reddish-purple birthmark type of blemish ("port wine stain") on the affected area of the leg. Patients with this condition may have bone and soft tissue overgrowth in the affected leg, and the leg may be abnormally long. Impressively large varicose veins may also be present. These patients are at high risk for pain, swelling, and possible blood-clot or bleeding complications.

There currently is no known cure for this syndrome, so specialists will usually work with patients and families to reduce the degree of symptoms and the risk of complications. Some of the exciting new techniques discussed in this book for treating varicose and spider vein disease and chronic venous insufficiency—including endovenous thermal ablation techniques and foam sclerotherapy injection, in tandem with either broadband intense pulse light or topical skin surface laser techniques—have been used to treat Klippel-Trenaunay Syndrome. They can help to reduce symptoms, prevent complications, and alleviate the neurovascular abnormalities on the skin's surface.

Because KTS is so rare—I have seen it only a couple of times in my career—very few vein specialists or vascular surgeons have experience treating it. I believe that patients with this condition should be referred to specialized health facilities, such as tertiary university hospital centers, where the physicians are better prepared to deal with it.

Pelvic Congestion Syndrome (PCS)

PCS affects young women of childbearing age, causing pain, pressure, or heaviness in the lower abdominal and pelvic regions. Painful varicose veins may also occur in the lower abdomen, groin, vulva, vagina, and upper thigh areas. Patients might also experience abnormal menstrual bleeding or vaginal discharge. The symptoms often will occur during late pregnancy. They can be more severe before menses, during periods of prolonged standing or sitting, or following sexual intercourse.

The nature of PCS is not well understood, but it seems to be related to the development of varicose veins and/or high venous pressure in the pelvic and ovarian veins within the lower abdominal and pelvic regions. Sometimes this condition, which often worsens during late pregnancy, is either completely or partially resolved after delivery. However, residual symptoms such as backaches, lethargy, and depression persist in some patients well after delivery.

Diagnosing PCS is tricky because similar symptoms can be caused by endometriosis, pelvic adhesions (scar tissue), a uterine fibroid tumor, or other gynecologic conditions.

Patients with the symptoms of PCS should work with their gynecologists to rule out other gynecologic or lower abdominal and pelvic conditions. Additional steps toward diagnosis might include having laparoscopic surgery, which is done using a scope and small incisions.

If the condition is caused by varicose veins or reflux in the ovarian veins due to leaking valves, it can often be diagnosed with magnetic resonance imaging (MRI) or with a contrast venogram x-ray, which is done through a catheter placed via a groin vein.

If PCS is diagnosed or strongly suspected, an interventional radiologist can often do what is called an embolization procedure, in which foam medication, coils, or small mechanical devices are placed through a catheter into the targeted offending pelvic or ovarian veins. This will seal the veins and reduce the abnormally high vein pressures.

When PCS is correctly diagnosed and treated, the patient has a high probability of symptom improvement. Medical reports indicate that some types of medical therapy, such as the use of temporary steroids or antidepressant-type medications, can relieve some symptoms and pain. Vein specialists can often successfully treat the varicose veins that may occur in the groin, vulvar, and upper thigh regions using foam medication injection. Microphlebectomy minor surgery can be performed on extraordinarily large veins, but I rarely find this necessary.

Venous Professional Organizations

Below are some of the major organizations that support the practice of phlebology. This information could be helpful to you for learning more about vein disease and finding a qualified physician. I recommend visiting these websites because they have excellent patient-education information.

- **The American Venous Forum (AVF)** is a quality organization with a membership made up of vascular surgeons and physicians who specialize in the treatment of vein disease. Many of AVF's members are affiliated with university medical centers. AVF's website (www.veinforum.org) is an excellent resource for finding qualified vein specialists. The patient section of veinforum.org is the best online patient resource I have found. Among other materials, it provides an excellent online book, *The Layman's Handbook of Venous Disorders*.

- **Vein Affiliates** is a network of board-certified surgeons throughout the United States who specialize or subspecialize in treating vein disease. The founder of the organization, Dr. Ron Bush of Cincinnati and Dayton, Ohio, is one of the pioneers in the field and one of the early and most prolific educators regarding state-of-the-art techniques for treating vein diseases. He was my most important mentor as I learned about the exciting, new venous techniques.

  The organization's website, www.veinaffiliates.com, lists a large number of qualified practitioners, many of whom I know personally. This is the resource I most highly recommend to patients who are looking for a qualified vein specialist.

- **The American College of Phlebology (ACP)** champions the treatment of vein disease as an emerging specialty. It devotes considerable energy to advancing training, research, and scientific development in the field. Membership is evidence of a commitment to, or at least an interest in, advancing the organization's goals.

  If you're seeking treatment for vein disease, you might want to visit this organization's website (www.phlebology.org) to find the names of member physicians in your area. However, I should caution you that members of ACP have widely varying levels of training, experience, and qualification. The ACP also has a website for patients and the public (www.healthyveins.org).

- **The American Board of Phlebology (ABPh)** held its first board-certification exam in 2008, at which time it certified the first 256 diplomates worldwide. I was proud to be among them. The board seeks to improve the standards of doctors and the quality of patient care with regard to vein disease.

  This organization's website (www.americanboardofphlebology.org) is an excellent resource for patients who want to find a vein practitioner in their area. To become a member of this organization, a physician must pass a rigorous examination and have a minimal level of documented clinical experience. This should be reassuring to patients who are looking for highly qualified physicians. The ACP and the ABPh have a positive, collaborative relationship.

- **International Union of Phlebology (UIP)** is an international organization that seeks to unite and organize venous societies from different countries. It may be helpful to those outside the United States. Their website is www.uip-phlebologyonline.org.

- **VeinDirectory.org** is a commercial organization that provides information about physicians throughout the United States who specialize in vein medicine. Physicians and vein-center practices pay to be listed on this website. Patient education sections are available.

- **Venous Disease Coalition** is a consortium of professional organizations and societies interested in scientific research and education related to venous disease. Their website, www.venousdiseasecoalition.org, provides an excellent patient education section for professionals and the public.

Suppliers of Compression Hosiery and Devices

LISTED BELOW ARE SOME OF THE LEADING SUPPLIERS OF COMPRESSION HOSE and other devices useful for conservative treatment of leg-vein problems. Some of these company websites have patient sections with educational material on leg compression therapy and leg-vein disease in general.

Sigvaris
Sigvaris, Inc.
1119 Highway 74 South
Peachtree City, GA 30269
800.322.7744
www.sigvarisusa.com

Jobst
BSN Medical Inc.
5825 Carnegie Blvd.
Charlotte, NC 28209-4633
704.554.9933
www.jobst-usa.com

Carolon

Carolon Company
601 Forum Pkwy., PO Box 1329
Rural Hall, NC 27045
800.334.0414
www.carolon.com

Ames Walker

Ames Walker Support Hosiery
856 Route 206, Suite 10 B
Hillsborough, NJ 08844
866.232.3655
www.ameswalker.com

medi

medi USA
6481 Franz Warner Parkway
PO Box 3000
Whitsett, NC 27377
800.633.6334
www.medi.usa.com

Juzo

PO Box 1088
Cuyahoga Falls, OH 44223
800.222.4999
www.juzousa.com

Gloria

Gloria Med USA
1107 Fair Oaks Avenue #462
South Pasadena, CA 91030
877.390.5347
www.GloriamedUSA.com

Venosan

Venosan North America
300 Industrial Park Avenue
PO Box 1067
Asheboro, NC 27204
800.432.5347
www.venosanusa.com

Total Vein Systems

901 Yale Street
Houston, TX 77008
888.868.8346
www.totalvein.com

CircAid

800.247.2243
www.circaid.com

Lympha Press

Lympha Press USA
232 Park Ave.
Manalapan, NJ 07726
888.596.7421
www.lympha-press.com

Suppliers of Vein Treatment Devices

BELOW ARE LISTED SOME OF THE LEADING COMPANIES THAT MARKET treatment devices for varicose and spider veins. Many have excellent patient education sections on their websites. Some feature photograph galleries and video demonstrations of treatment techniques.

Dornier
Dornier MedTech America, Inc.
1155 Roberts Boulevard
Kennesaw, GA 30144
800.367.6437
www.dornier.com

Cool Touch
Cool Touch, Inc.
9085 Foothills Boulevard
Roseville, CA 95747
877.858.2665
www.cooltouch.com

AngioDynamics
AngioDynamics, Inc.
603 Queensbury Ave.
Queensbury, NY 12804
800.772.6446
www.VenaCure-ELVT.com

Covidien VNUS
VNUS Medical Technologies, Inc.
5799 Fontenoso Way
San Jose, CA 95138
888.797.8346
www.vnus.com

Sciton

Sciton, Inc.
925 Commercial Street
Palo Alto, CA 94303
888.646.6999
http://.sciton.com

VeinGogh Ohmic Thermolysis System

Refine USA, LLC
340 3rd Ave. S., Suite C
Jacksonville Beach, FL 32250
866.333.6858
www.refineusa.com

Veinwave

Veinwave USA
567 47th Ave.
San Francisco, CA 94121
888.902.7876
www.veinwave.com

Total Vein Systems

901 Gail St.
Houston, TX 77008
888.868.8346
www.totalvein.com

Index

About the Author

DR. GREG MARTIN IS A GENERAL SURGEON CERTIFIED BY THE AMERICAN Board of Surgery and the American Board of Phlebology. He earned his Doctor of Medicine degree at the Medical University of South Carolina and fulfilled his residency and internship requirements at Northwestern University in Chicago. He currently operates vein treatment centers at the following locations:

Coastal Georgia Vein Center
650 Scranton Road, Suite C
Brunswick, GA 31520
912.267.9550
www.CoastalVeins.net

South Georgia Vein Center
3338 Country Club Road, Suite M
Valdosta, GA 31605
229.259.9666
www.ValdostaVeins.net

GREGORY D. MARTIN, FACS
Fellow, American College of Surgeons
American College of Phlebology
American Board of Surgery
American Board of Phlebology
RVT (Registered Vascular Ultrasound Technician, ADDMS)
RPVI (Registered Physician in Vascular Interpretation, ARDMS)

How to Order Copies of This Book

Distributed in the United States of America by

Narrow Gate Books
2110 Slaughter Lane #110
PMB 417
Austin, TX 78748
PHONE: 512.669.5744
FAX: 512.904.8120
Email: *info@narrowgatebooks.com*
Website: *www.narrowgatebooks.com*

Quantity discounts are available.

Order online at:
www.GregMartinMD.com/book.html

Plentiful Publishing
650 Scranton Road, Suite C
Brunswick, GA 31520
Phone: 800.276.1903
Email: *info@plentifulpublishing.com*

How to Order Promotional Copies of this Book

Discounted prices • Minimum order 100 copies

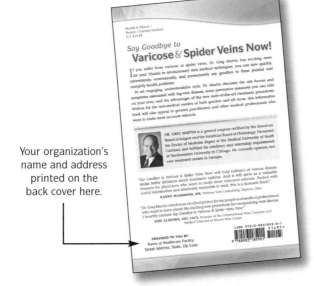

Your organization's name and address printed on the back cover here.

For information and pricing, contact

Plentiful Publishing
800.276.1903 • *info@plentifulpublishing.com*